Praise for The Hidden Link between Vision and Learning

"This book is a terrific introduction to children's vision. It considers vision and visual problems much more fully than is customary and in a way that parents and educators can easily understand. Moreover, it discusses vision as it occurs in the whole child—a living, breathing, thinking, feeling child who is coping with the real world. As such, the book makes a valuable contribution to the child development literature." —**William Crain**, professor of psychology, City College of New York; author of *Theories of Development: Concepts and Applications*

"When Wendy Rosen couldn't figure out why her bright, eager-to-learn daughter was struggling in elementary school, she set out to find answers. And find them she did: in a little-diagnosed and little-understood vision-related learning problem that affects an untold number of other children as well. In The Hidden Link Between Vision and Learning, Rosen brings her parental love and determination, as well as her teacher knowledge and experience, to the lucky ones who will benefit from her research, her stories, and her advice." —**Sara Bennett**, coauthor of *The Case Against Homework*; founder, Stop Homework

"Wendy Beth Rosen has written a fascinating and important book on a topic too often overlooked: the connection between vision and learning. I certainly didn't know that there is a difference between vision and eyesight, that there's more to vision than 20/20, or that millions of children struggle in school due to undiagnosed vision problems. Parents and teachers alike need to read this eye-opening book!" —**Rae Pica**, author of *What If Everybody Understood Child Development?*

"Written by an education consultant, this marvelous book offers unique insights on why the association between vision and learning has remained hidden. More than a commentary on a system that has failed our children, Ms. Rosen's diligent research and accessible prose will benefit countless numbers of parents and educators." —**Leonard J. Press**, OD, FAAO, FCOVD, optometric director, The Vision and Learning Center

THE HIDDEN LINK BETWEEN VISION AND LEARNING

Why Millions of Learning-Disabled Children Are Misdiagnosed

Wendy Beth Rosen

ROWMAN & LITTLEFIELD
Lanham • Boulder • New York • London

Published by Rowman & Littlefield
A wholly owned subsidiary of The Rowman & Littlefield Publishing Group,
Inc.
4501 Forbes Boulevard, Suite 200, Lanham, Maryland 20706
www.rowman.com

Unit A, Whitacre Mews, 26-34 Stannary Street, London SE11 4AB

British Library Cataloguing in Publication Information Available

Library of Congress Cataloging-in-Publication Data

Names: Rosen, Wendy Beth, 1965–
Title: The hidden link between vision and learning : why millions of learning-disabled children are
    misdiagnosed / Wendy Beth Rosen.
Description: Lanham, Maryland : Rowman and Littlefield, 2016. | Includes bibliographical refer-
    ences and index.
Identifiers: LCCN 2015043393 (print) | LCCN 2015044932 (ebook) | ISBN 9781475813135
    (cloth : alk. paper) | ISBN 9781475813159 (electronic)
Subjects: LCSH: Children with visual disabilities–Education. | Vision disorders in chil-
    dren–Diagnosis.
Classification: LCC HV1626 .R68 2016 | DDC 371.91/1–dc23 LC record available at http://
    lccn.loc.gov/2015043393

Printed in the United States of America

For Sara and Jonah, with immeasurable love.

And for every child everywhere, so that you may realize your full potential and be your best self.

"Never doubt that a small group of thoughtful, committed citizens can change the world; indeed, it's the only thing that ever has."—Margaret Mead

CONTENTS

FOREWORD

I have had the pleasure to come to know Wendy Beth Rosen as a vision therapy parent, as an educational consultant, and now as an author. She has always been an inquisitive, intelligent, and extremely dedicated parent and vision therapy advocate. Once she saw the striking improvement in learning capability and performance of her own children after vision therapy, she became quite concerned that so few parents and educators had even heard about the connection between vision and learning. I have seen this response many times before, especially with parents of my patients who have completed a vision therapy program. I often try to give them suggestions of how they can raise awareness in their local schools, PTA organizations, and communities.

When Wendy informed me that she wanted to write a book about vision-related learning problems, I was pleased but privately incredulous. How would a nonoptometric person be able to understand and communicate this fairly complex topic? Two years later, when I finally read the manuscript, I was "blown away." Wendy has done an incredible job of explaining the critical connection between vision and learning in a way that is interesting, scientifically accurate, and compelling. I am certain that parents, patients, educators, and other interested professionals will come away with a much deeper sense of understanding and, even more importantly, a desire to do something about the lack of proper screening and referral for treatment for these often very treatable visual conditions.

I will be recommending this book for vision therapy parents, patients, educators, and others for an in-depth but very readable treatise on vision-related learning problems and what can be done to solve them. I am convinced that this book will make an important difference and eventually help many children and others who will benefit from this knowledge.

Barry Tannen, OD, FCOVD, FAAO
Board Certified in Vision Therapy and Development
EyeCare Professionals, PC

PREFACE

One in four school-age children have an undetected vision problem that can interfere with their ability to learn.[1] This can impact a range of learners from the bright underachiever to the student with moderate to severe learning difficulties.

Many children have their visual acuity screened annually in school, but this test only checks their distance eyesight. This "20/20" measurement only tells us how well someone sees at a distance of twenty feet. Vision actually comprises more than a dozen different skills that enable the brain to process visual input coming in through the eyes, making it possible for us to successfully navigate through the world. Some of these lesser-known vision skills include eye movement control, visual memory, eye teaming, and visual closure, to name just a few. If these skills are not present, or are not working optimally, a child cannot perform up to his or her potential.

At the present time, visual skills are not routinely and comprehensively examined to determine if a deficit is present and interfering with a child's capacity for learning. Consequently, we are missing critical information about a child's readiness for school. Beyond this lies the alarming fact that many symptoms of visual deficits can mimic those of dyslexia and AD/HD. There are, as a result, countless numbers of children who are classified as special education students or are medicated, or both, who may be wrongly diagnosed.

I know how this impacts a child's life. My daughter, Sara, was diagnosed with several visual deficits that interfered with her academic performance and attention span. Fortunately for her, we were referred to a doctor who was familiar with vision-related learning problems. This was sheer luck, as we found out years later.

We saw the first signs in second grade. For the first time, we noticed that Sara seemed stressed about school. This was unusual, as Sara had always loved school. Class work was starting to come home unfinished, with little notes written at the top of the page by the teacher asking for it to be completed for homework. Her handwriting, we noticed, was better in kindergarten. We were discouraged to see this skill declining in its development. A lack of motivation, we thought? Then there was our first parent-teacher conference in the fall. We walked in and sat down at the table with her teacher, knowing what our agenda would include.

"You know what I'm going to say," she began. We did. Apparently she had the same agenda, and so began our journey, though we did not yet know it at the time. We all agreed that Sara had a difficult time staying focused on her work. She was bright and capable and loved to learn, but this problem was slowing her down and getting in the way of her ability to keep up with her class work. Behavior modification strategies, including stickers, self-check charts, and a clock on her desk, helped Sara plod through the rest of the year and helped her to complete her work somewhat more efficiently. Still, in the back of our minds burned the question of why she had to work so hard at this.

The following year, from the first day Sara entered third grade, it seemed as if she had been pulled under by a big wave. There were new demands and more work, and by November we all felt as if Sara had hit a wall. Although she understood the material, Sara was more frustrated and stressed than ever. It was painful to watch her struggle so much.

Unable to figure out why Sara was having such a hard time, we decided to go through the child study team evaluation process to see if, perhaps, there was a hidden learning issue that was not readily identifiable in the classroom. We also wondered if Sara had AD/HD since she exhibited such a hard time staying focused.

The results of the evaluation showed that Sara scored in the average to high average range in all academic areas, except one. She fell below grade level in written expression. All her other academic scores as well as her IQ scores were also in the normal range, except for one. This test measured her ability to comprehend and repeat a pattern of symbols, and she scored disproportionately lower on this test than all the others.

Ultimately, the child study team could not explain why Sara was struggling so much, and we didn't have any new insight as a result of the process. All we knew was that Sara qualified for extra help with her writing, which of course we agreed to, since we wanted to do all we could to help her.

Still wanting more in the way of an explanation, however, we followed up with another psychologist to get a second opinion. When we shared Sara's evaluation with her, she immediately saw a connection between the low patterning score and Sara's writing deficiency. She explained to us that these two indicators were significant and suggested that she might have a visual issue that needed to be addressed.

When she applied these scores to a formula that measured for this potential problem and Sara's score fell out of the normal range, her concern was confirmed. I then mentioned that we were planning to take Sara to the eye doctor to see if maybe she needed glasses because she had been complaining of frequent headaches.

Taking all of this into account, it was recommended that we take Sara to see a behavioral optometrist. We had never heard of this kind of doctor before, also sometimes referred to as a developmental optometrist. This specialist, we were told, uses special diagnostic measures that go beyond a regular eye exam to identify and diagnose visual deficiencies.

The outcome of her initial exam was astounding. We learned that Sara had 20/20 eyesight, but it was discovered that she had a visual disorder called convergence insufficiency (CI). CI is a disorder whereby the eyes do not work as a team, as they are supposed to in normal binocular vision. Rather than focusing on one image at the same time, Sara's eyes were focusing on two different places, consequently sending conflicting messages to the brain.

In other words, Sara was seeing double.

A follow-up comprehensive visual and perceptual examination showed that Sara was deficient in a number of other areas as well. These areas included eye movement control, which affects how well a child can track along the lines of print on a page; visual motor integration, which impacts handwriting and written expression (which explained her evaluation results); and focus accommodation, which manifests itself in a child's ability to adjust his or her focus from near to far distances smoothly.

All the while we had been saying that Sara seemed to have a hard time staying focused on her work, and it turned out that she, in fact, literally had a problem focusing her eyes!

The good news was that these disorders could be corrected permanently through vision therapy. Vision therapy, we learned, is a process that helps to retrain the eyes and the brain to process visual information correctly and helps children with disorders such as these. It is effective in over 90 percent of cases. In Sara's case, the prognosis was excellent, as long as she worked hard at it.

She did. Once a week Sara spent an hour with a vision therapist doing a range of activities that helped her eyes and brain to relearn how to process visual input correctly. In addition, I was required to work with her daily at home for about twenty minutes on a regimen that supported the work Sara was doing in the office. At the time, this was a big commitment for both of us.

No matter how often I reflect on this experience, I will never have enough words to adequately sum up its worth. The first day I did vision therapy with Sara I was amazed to discover that I could actually see how her eyes worked. I could see how both eyes were functioning differently and how she struggled with the activity because of this.

Sara also began to wear glasses for close-up work to help relieve the stress she felt when she tried to focus on anything within arm's length. Since she could focus on the chalkboard fine but couldn't shift well to near-point distances, she wore a bifocal. The top part of the lens was normal, but the bottom part made everything look like it was further away so her eyes didn't have to work so hard. This brought her some relief in the meantime while we worked every day on helping her ocular muscles get stronger.

It was not easy. There were days we both grumbled through the exercises, days when Sara didn't have the energy or just would have rather been doing something else. Yet I saw how hard she worked despite the many difficult challenges she was meeting both physically and mentally. Remarkably I watched my daughter in awe at times, at what she was accomplishing, and I deeply admired her determination.

Nine months later, Sara graduated from vision therapy. Her checkpoints throughout the process indicated that she was progressing beautifully, but the enormity of that moment, signifying how far she had come, was felt by both of us when the staff presented Sara with her diploma and we both cried.

Sara scored readings in the teens on her initial vision assessments and finished with scores in the nineties. The best part, however, was that Sara was so proud of all that she accomplished and, in addition to her vision skills improving greatly, her confidence soared. Sara was subsequently declassified and no longer needed the special services that were provided to her by the school. Best of all, she went on to thrive in all facets of learning.

As parents, we were profoundly grateful that we had gotten to the root of Sara's struggles and relieved to see her problems resolve. I believe that Sara knew what she was capable of all along, and her inability to realize this was partly the source of her frustration. I think this is the case for many children.

As a teacher, I had worked closely with child study teams to address many learning issues in my own students, yet I had never heard of vision-related learning problems. A whole new world had opened up for me, and I felt like shouting about it from the rooftops. I felt incredibly fortunate that we had stumbled onto a professional equipped with this knowledge.

I also realized that not everyone is so lucky, and that there must be untold numbers of kids out there who are not being helped. If parents, teachers, pediatricians, and therapists are made aware of this knowledge, many hidden vision problems may be caught and lives turned around. We can hear when a child exhibits a speech problem, but we have no way of knowing how the world looks to a child with a vision problem.

Furthermore, children don't usually realize that they have a vision problem. They, in their innocence, think that everyone sees the way they do. When Sara told us some time into the therapy process that the words on the page didn't look 3-D anymore, we were speechless. We were astonished to learn that this was how the text looked to her when she read.

Learning about this changed not only my daughter's life, but my life as well. I became passionately inspired and embarked on a mission to get the word out so that other kids who are struggling with hidden visual disorders could be recognized and helped. I have seen evidence of it firsthand. I understand how this knowledge can be the key to a child's success and have dedicated myself to educating others about it. You are holding the capstone to a decade of my research, experience, outreach, and hope.

Herein lies the purpose of this book. This is a subject that has far-reaching personal and societal ramifications once understood and recognized for its inherent potential to turn struggling lives around. The unique aspect to *The Hidden Link Between Vision and Learning* is the perspective I'm able to bring to this subject through firsthand experience from two key vantage points: that of a parent as well as a teacher. Having been immersed on both sides, I have observed and learned a great deal about how these hidden disorders play out for a child.

Additionally, I have spoken with countless parents who have also gone through it and who share their perspectives in a special section devoted to their personal stories. Perhaps they will resonate with you.

With so many children struggling with learning and behavior issues, and so many schools struggling to meet these needs and so often falling short, this book will speak to, literally, millions. It is my hope that in offering a user-friendly resource that conveys this research-backed knowledge to the general population, parents and educators will be able to find the missing piece to the puzzle. The world has never been more ready for this information and insight and the potential answers that it could provide for so many. This knowledge will change children's lives.

INTRODUCTION

Metaphorically speaking, we will be both nearsighted and farsighted throughout these pages. This book begins with a close-up look at what vision is. We will then look out into the distance at the big picture to understand the far-reaching effects vision has on our experiences, and that our experiences in turn have on our vision.

Most importantly, the knowledge that lies between the covers of this book will potentially offer answers and help for the inestimable numbers of children who are struggling with learning. This will be tendered through carefully unfolding an overview of several fields whose influence intersect with profound significance, beginning with one that many people have never heard about.

Behavioral optometry and developmental optometry are essentially one and the same field. This specialty branch of optometry holds the key for unlocking the potential of many children. The term *behavioral* was first conceived to highlight the effects that behavior can have on visual development. Recognizing that there are many, many variables that also factor into visual development, the term *developmental* was later adopted to reflect this. I use these two titles interchangeably throughout this book. Further explanation of the nuances behind the origins of these transposable terms awaits you.

Some books can be read piecemeal, with chapters bearing self-contained portions of information that can be assimilated into your psyche according to your own agenda.

This is not one of those books.

You will want to start at the beginning and read this book chapter by chapter, as each one builds on the previous with specialized knowledge that you will need in order to understand what comes next.

The beginning chapters will equip you with an in-depth explanation of what vision really is, how it steers our lives, and what the effects of its dysfunction can look like. This information will broaden your perspective immensely, enabling you to perceive just how important this sense is to the process of learning and even to the quality of life. What's more, you will be able to associate specific symptoms with observable behaviors in the children you care for and begin to uncover why they may be struggling with an unrecognized vision disorder.

The information in this book will not enable you to diagnose a child with a vision disorder. Only a behavioral or developmental optometrist can do this. However, the knowledge you are about to gain can help you discern if there are indicators that warrant an examination with one of these specialists.

You may be wondering, "Why isn't this common knowledge since it affects so many children?" Like you, I had the same question. It is a good question and a very important one. My work in this area grew out of this question and many others, most especially, "Why is my daughter struggling so much?"

I've taught my students and my own children that asking questions is one of the smartest things you can do. People ask many questions about this specialized field, and some of them challenge its efficacy. Fortunately, many responses portray behavioral optometry in its rightful light, as a profession that treats vision problems that affect learning and behavior. Unfortunately, other responses misguidedly invalidate its value and success. Myths have grown out of this disparagement, and potentially helpful treatment has been avoided because of this.

We will dive into these necessary and essential questions, and with a newly acquired, deeper working knowledge of vision and its all-encompassing influence, you will process explanations that will continue to expand your increasing measure of understanding. First and foremost, however, this elucidation will also set the record straight and enable you to embrace this knowledge with assurance and confidence. As you will soon discover, the impact of vision on individuals and community is not only leaps and bounds beyond what most realize, but is also highly underrated.

Conversely, the impact of our cultural ways on vision and its development, especially in very young children, is also largely unrecognized and undervalued and will be explored in great depth. As we contemplate the educational climate we have sanctioned, its outcomes and intentions will be questioned and examined. Additionally, we will delve into the connection between vision and topics such as health and wellness, crime, and educational policy.

There are many inspiring stories out in the world that tell of progressive work being done to foster a true, comprehensive interpretation of what vision is. This understanding is far from familiar to most and needs to become commonplace. Moving personal anecdotes telling how children went from failure to success and about groundbreaking actions taken by dedicated professionals will drive home this need.

Knowledge and awareness are powerful tools for change. You will be well equipped by the end of this book to effect change in individual lives, and perhaps even a little piece of the world.

THE DIFFERENCE BETWEEN VISION AND EYESIGHT

There is a story about a man who unfortunately lost his sight when he was a toddler. Through a remarkable surgical procedure, however, his sight was restored to him in his thirties. After removing the bandages to see if the surgery was successful, his doctor did the following exercise with him.

Holding up a picture of a cylinder, he asked his patient a number of questions about it, including whether he could identify it. It was determined that his eyesight had indeed been restored and that he could physically *see* the picture in front of him; however, he did not know what it was that he was looking at.

He had to learn that the parallel vertical lines and the elliptical shapes coordinated in a certain way to create what is called a cylinder. He had to make the connection between what his eyes were seeing and what his brain was now learning about the object. This latter process is what we call vision. Eyesight is the physiological ability to receive input through the eyes. Vision is the ability to understand what the input is.[1]

Try this exercise. Presented here is an image of a familiar object. See if you can make out what it is.

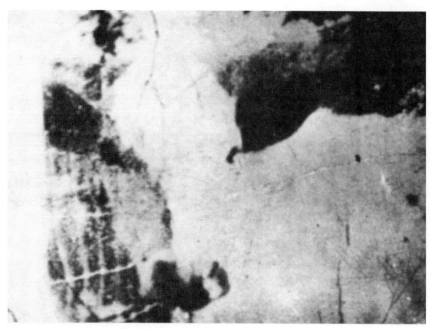

Figure I.I. **"What Is It?"** *Photo courtesy of the Optometric Extension Program*
Foundation

Did you see a cow? If not, don't worry. It's meant to be almost indiscernible, to prove a point. Now that you know what it is, you can go back and look at it again and be able to make sense of the lines, shapes, and shadows to perceive that it is, indeed, a cow. Your brain will assimilate all the previous knowledge you have about what cows look like with the visual input coming in through your eyes to make sense of what you're seeing. What's more, if you try to go back and see the picture as an amorphous composite of black, white, and gray tones, you likely will have a hard time *not* seeing the cow. This is because you went from using your eyesight to acquiring vision.

When children have their eyes screened in the school nurse's office or at the pediatrician's office, parents come away with a reading that is in a range of 20/20 or some variation of this. Based on this reading, parents feel they know how their child is functioning visually. Why would parents think otherwise? Children have been tested with this method since 1862! That is when the Snellen chart, named after its creator, Dr. Herman Snellen, a Dutch ophthalmologist, came into use.[2]

Over a century and a half later, it is still the primary tool used despite major discoveries in how the visual system works and how we subsequently need to evaluate it accordingly. Yet this method only identifies a mere 5 *percent* of vision problems in children.

The Snellen chart tests for visual acuity. Visual acuity can be defined as how clear symbols or objects look at a certain distance. This is useful information, but it only tells us a fraction of the whole story. Pediatricians, school nurses, and parents come away with an understanding of how well a child sees at a distance of twenty feet. Period. What isn't known is how well a child can see at a distance of ten feet, five feet, or within an even closer range such as two or three feet—where most schoolwork is done. It does not evaluate eye health or the rest of a child's visual story.

Beyond acuity, there are many visual skills that allow us to successfully find our way in the world. They work in concert with the other sensory systems. We rely on our senses to help us move through life. In this view lies a simple but fundamental fact: our bodies are designed to move.[3] Every function of the body that involves movement has a purpose behind it. This can be said for obvious actions, like walking, to more subtle movements, like blinking and breathing.

The physiological act of blinking serves several purposes. It helps lubricate the eyes and fends off any dust that may cause irritation. Plus, it gives our eyes momentary breaks from focusing. Try focusing on this text for a few moments without blinking, and you will feel how necessary this involuntary movement is. Each time we blink, our eyes close for three-tenths of a second. That adds up to a total of thirty minutes a day that our eyes involuntarily close for cleansing and rest.[4]

Breathing needs no explanation; however, many of us walk around unaware that we are not breathing correctly. In order for our blood, and therefore our whole body, to be optimally oxygenated, we should be inhaling deeply, so that our lungs fully expand and the air goes into the deep part of the lobes. Often, we take shallow breaths, which is not ideal.

Try this exercise. Place your hand on your belly. If you are breathing correctly, you should feel your abdomen gently rising and falling with each complete breath.[5] If this is not happening, chances are you will instead notice your chest and shoulders moving up and down, meaning that you are not breathing fully. In our fast-paced, 24/7 lifestyle, we can feel out of breath at times. It's because we are! We need to give the life-sustaining and nourishing act of breathing more attention. It is one of the most precious and essential ways we can care for ourselves.

Our eyes are designed to move as well. Vision is a highly complex process that involves subtle eye movements of which we are usually not even aware. These movements coordinate with the neurological system and allow us to accurately understand what comes into our view and to interact with the world around us. If the eyes are not moving properly, or if the wiring in the vision center of the brain is faulty, we will not be able to perceive visual input correctly.

There are more than a dozen visual skills that incorporate subtle forms of movement within the eyes and the eye muscles and that coordinate with other movement systems of the body. These skills affect how well we function and perform in all areas of our lives but are especially critical to a child's overall developmental process, and especially academic achievement. These skills are not evaluated in the vision screening that utilizes only the Snellen chart and often go unchecked.

A comprehensive eye exam is less common than a vision screening and greatly differs from a screening in that it encompasses an in-depth evaluation of all these visual skills, as well as eye health. The American Optometric Association recommends that this exam be done first at six months of age, then at three years, and again just before entering kindergarten. After that, yearly checkups are recommended to make sure vision is developing normally.[6] If it is not, catching any deficits early in these foundational years can alleviate much frustration, struggle, and stress for a child down the road. Yet only 14 percent of children are getting this type of exam by the time they enter first grade, according to the Better Vision Institute.[7]

In order to fully understand and appreciate how vision impacts our everyday lives, refer to the comprehensive list of vision skills in the textbox that follows, complete with definitions and examples. This will be instrumental in helping you understand how deficits in any of these areas can affect a child's learning capacity, which we will explore in greater depth in the next chapter.

Visual Acuity is the measurement of how clearly we see at certain distances. This ability may be influenced by certain existing conditions, such as nearsightedness, farsightedness, and astigmatism. All of these conditions are very common and correctable with eyeglasses or contact lenses.

Nearsightedness (myopia) occurs when we can see objects clearly up close but not far away.

Farsightedness (hyperopia) requires greater focusing demand the closer a target is to us, causing fatigue. With low amounts of farsightedness, we can still see objects clearly at distance and at near.

Astigmatism is a condition whereby vision can be blurred at any distance. This happens when the cornea or the lens inside the eye has an irregular shape to its curvature, making it difficult for light to fully reach the retina in one meridian to allow for proper focusing. Astigmatism can be present in conjunction with nearsightedness or farsightedness.

Certain eye diseases can also impact visual acuity.

Having 20/20 vision means that we can see clearly at 20 feet what is supposed to be seen clearly at this distance. If you're told that you have, for example, 20/60 vision, it means that you have to be 20 feet from what a person with normal vision can see at 60 feet.

An acuity problem is why many people will be prescribed corrective eyewear. Lenses are specially designed to bend the light so that it comes into the eye and reaches the retina precisely as it should so that images can be seen clearly. With routine checkups to adjust the prescription for any changes in acuity that may occur over time, eyeglasses or contact lenses can keep someone with an acuity problem comfortable and seeing clearly without interference in his or her daily activities. More than half the population of the United States use some form of compensatory lenses.

Eye Movement Control, also known as *oculomotility*, determines how well the eyes move together. It enables us to track along a line of print, track a moving target such as a ball, and adjust our focus from near distances to far distances smoothly and efficiently. This movement is dependent upon the efficiency, flexibility, endurance, and health of the eye muscles.

Being able to move our eyes efficiently is a necessary skill that involves speed, control, and accuracy. This skill comes into play crucially in the classroom, where children are required to constantly pay attention to information that is coming to them from multiple sources and distances.

Vergence is the ability to move our eyes together to focus on a certain point.

The inward movement of the eyes to focus on an object at a close distance is called *convergence*. If you hold up your finger in front of your nose at a moderate distance, then move it closer and stay focused on it, your eyes will converge to keep it as one image. The eyes will have a cross-eyed appearance while doing this. Outward movement of the eyes while looking off into the distance is called *divergence*.

Eye Teaming, also called *binocularity*, consists of the ability for each eye to send information to the brain and for the brain to put the information together so that we can have one clear image. Each eye functions independently and sees the world slightly differently, which is normal. Binocularity is a sensory process that fuses the information and works in concert with vergence. The information coming into the brain from the input received through each eye is created into a 3-D image that enables us to judge depth, understand relationships, and grasp spatial awareness.

If the eyes are not working as a team, this can result in blurred, scrambled, or moving print; problems with depth perception; and double vision. Stress on this part of the visual system can lead to confusion, difficulty concentrating, eyestrain, and frustration. When this overload becomes too difficult for the brain to handle, the brain will sometimes disregard some of the information coming in through one eye, causing what is called *suppression*. This can greatly reduce the amount of information the brain is able to understand and retain and can cause confusion.

Focus Accommodation is the capacity to efficiently and quickly change and adjust our focus from near to far distances, such as from a book in front of us to a chalkboard or whiteboard. It should feel effortless to sustain this focus for extended periods of time at any distance. How well our eyes can accommodate our focusing needs will depend on how much power, or stamina, we have.

Depth Perception is the ability to see the world three-dimensionally by perceiving width, depth, and height. Our eyes coordinate the separate images coming in to create a 3-D image, allowing us to understand how far away something is.

Peripheral Vision allows you to see what is not directly in front of you without turning your head. We are able to see directly ahead while simultaneously taking in information about what is happening on either side of us, as well as above and below eye level. Peripheral vision enables us to move through space smoothly. It also helps us keep our place by guiding us as we track along a line of print. If our peripheral vision is not functioning properly, we may only be able to focus on a few words at a time. Under these circumstances, sometimes referred to as "tunnel vision," our reading efficiency is reduced.

Visual Spatial Skills is a broad term delineating the various abilities that enable us to understand and navigate our place in the space we occupy. These skills are governed by the concepts of laterality and directionality.

Laterality is the awareness that there are two different sides to the body, left and right, which are separated by an invisible midline. In order to navigate comfortably and successfully in our surroundings, we first must be aware of and be comfortable in our own space—our body. This is where we learn the idea of "left" and "right," key concepts that we build on as we develop the capacity for physical coordination, balance, and cognition. Laterality awareness precedes the development of directionality.

Directionality is the understanding of up, down, in front, behind, or any combination of these. This skill is critical for decoding letters and reading. Being able to move the eyes efficiently is central to developing strong directionality abilities. This is an example of how our visual skills are integrated with the rest of our body.

Bilateral Integration is the ability to recognize the difference between the two sides of the body and coordinate them. These skills help us with movement and any activities that involve the use of both sides of the body in order to carry out a task.

Visual Spatial Relations allow us to differentiate between similar characteristics of an object or form. Proficiency with this enables us to develop problem-solving and higher-level thinking skills.

Visual Spatial Orientation is the ability to recognize left from right, up from down, and forward and backward, and apply this awareness to our bodily actions as we interact with the world around us.

Visual Motor Integration involves the facility to coordinate bodily movement with the information coming in through the eyes. These skills are often referred to as eye-body or eye-hand coordination. Information that comes in through the eyes is transmitted to the brain, which then dispatches our muscles to move a certain way so that we can complete a certain task, such as catching a ball, writing, and putting one foot in front of the other.

Visual Memory encompasses the ability to immediately remember characteristics of visually presented material.

Visual Spatial Memory is the ability to recognize specific features of objects or forms, their location in space, and their relationship to each other. It also involves the ability to reproduce a symbol or object in its entirety or any of its specific features. This skill comes into play when we create a mental picture of a lost object we are trying to find and when we see in our mind a picture that corresponds to a word we read. This skill is instrumental in helping children comprehend what they read, as well as in copying information off the board.

Visual Sequential Memory makes it possible for us to remember symbols or characters in the order in which they were seen. This skill is very important for spelling, remembering phone numbers, and recognizing patterns.

Figure Ground is the ability to simultaneously search for a specific form or object in a given context while dismissing surrounding unimportant information. We use this skill when we search for a specific object that we're looking for in a drawer or scanning a text to find specific information. This skill helps us to "not get lost in the details."

Visual Closure is the ability to visualize a complete image with only partial information about the whole. This skill allows us to read through material and understand its content quickly. We don't have to focus on every letter in a word to know what the word is. It enables us to be efficient readers and thinkers.

Visual Form Recognition/Discrimination involves the ability to identify distinguishing characteristics between similar forms or objects. This is significant in helping us differentiate between similarly spelled words like to/too, run/ran, and was/saw.

Visual Form Constancy is the ability to understand that the visual information about a form or object is consistent despite other variables that could affect its perception. This helps us recognize the constancy of an object despite changes, such as being able to recognize that the letter "b" makes the same sound whether it is lowercase or uppercase.

Visual Speed and Span of Perception is the pace at which content is being processed and the quantity able to be grasped.

Visualization enables us to picture an image in our mind's eye that we have seen before and to change this image through our own imagination, as well as the ability to create new images for ourselves.

Automaticity is a term used to describe the goal of all visual skills combined—for visual processing to become automatic, with minimal effort. This is central to efficient learning and optimal functioning.

Now, in just this short time, you have made a huge leap in your understanding of why vision is much more than 20/20! There are more than two dozen visual skills listed here.[8] That's a lot to grasp. To help you as we move through these next chapters, you may refer to the organized categories provided here in the following textbox that classify each skill in its larger domain. This should support your own visual memory as you begin to get a handle on the relationships between these skills and their effects on learning and behavior.

Please note that several skill areas overlap, and categorizing them is not a black-and-white business. Some skills can fall into more than one category. And some skills, you'll notice, are the sole inhabitants of their own category. If you do any Googling on this subject, you may run into this as you peruse other resources and find that something listed under one heading may be referred to under another someplace else. This is not in error; it simply reflects the interrelationships between skills.

CATEGORIES OF VISUAL SKILLS

Visual Acuity

Eye Movement Skills

- eye movement control (oculomotility)
- eye teaming (binocularity)
- vergence

Focus Accommodation

Depth Perception

Peripheral Vision

Visual Motor Integration

- gross-motor eye-body coordination
- fine-motor eye-body coordination

Visual Spatial Skills

- laterality
- directionality
- bilateral integration
- visual spatial relations
- visual spatial orientation

Vision Perception

- visualization
- visual form recognition/discrimination
- visual form constancy
- visual speed and span of perception
- visual memory
- visual sequential memory

- visual spatial memory
- visual closure
- figure ground

Automaticity

To fully grasp the profound role that vision plays in our day-to-day activities, consider this: 80 percent of the neurological pathways in the brain connect with the visual system. *Eighty percent!* The rest are home to all the other senses combined. We get an astounding amount of information about the world through vision. Clearly then, when one or more of these skills are not functioning as they should, it will thwart how well we can do any number of things.

When considering the interdependence of these skills and our reliance on them for optimal comfort and functioning, it's easy to understand why it's so critical to ensure that all facets of the visual system are up and running. It is even more compelling then to make sure we thoroughly examine all aspects of a child's vision so that if any deficits exist, they can be identified and corrected. How we do this makes all the difference, which underscores the importance of getting a comprehensive eye examination.

What's more, we are still discovering new information about the intricate systems deep in the brain that allow us to use our vision in ways that are not yet fully understood. Think about the expression "picture something in your mind's eye." What exactly is our mind's eye, and where is it located? How do we picture an image that we don't actually *see* in a physical sense?

Still, we "see" with our imagination all the time. With our eyes closed as we try to fall asleep at night, we may picture the events of our day, the faces of people we love, what the weather is doing outside, or any number of possibilities. This practice is called *visualization*.

Visualization may also be used as a tool for relaxation. Imagining a pristine forest, tropical beach, or country meadow filled with wildflowers can transport us to a serene setting in our mind that is thought to have beneficial effects not only on our mental state but on our physical state as well. There is much study being done about this, and scientists have many different views about the highly intricate neurological workings that interact with so many other processes that influence the human experience.

The findings of a 2008 research study out of Vanderbilt University showed that the mental imagery we visualize in "our mind's eye" can have a direct impact on our perception. Stating the difficulty in measuring the imagination due to its subjective nature, Joel Pearson, research associate in the Vanderbilt Department of Psychology and lead author of the study, notes: "This is the first research to definitively show that imagining something changes vision both while you are imagining it and later on." Further investigation in collaboration with coauthors Frank Tong, associate professor of psychology, and Colin Clifford of the University of Sydney brought these findings to light: "It has been very hard to pin down in the laboratory what exactly someone is experiencing when it comes to imagery, because it is so subjective," says Tong. "We found that the imagery effect, while found in all of our subjects, could differ a lot in strength across subjects. So this might give us a metric to measure the strength of mental imagery in individuals and how that imagery may influence perception. More recently, with advances in human brain imaging, we now know that when you imagine something parts of the visual brain do light up and you see activity there," says Pearson. "So there's more and more evidence suggesting that there is a huge overlap between mental imagery and seeing the same thing. Our work shows that not only are imagery and vision related, but imagery directly influences what we see."[9]

Here we have discernible evidence showing that what we visualize in our imagination forms a relationship with what we actually see in the world around us through our eyes. This is a very stirring concept and holds much promise for new discovery in its power and future application.

What we do have a firmly rooted understanding of now, though, is that chances for children to develop strong visualization skills are diminishing. Opportunities to exercise this skill are decreasing enormously with each hour of screen time that slips by. With very little, if any at all, left to the imagination, whether on a TV screen, computer screen, or iPhone, children are not using their creative imaginations. Yet visualization is important for both practical and aesthetic reasons.

Being able to find your way to and from destinations is one important application. Being swept away in your imagination to another place and time in a book is another. This timeless gift begins when we are read to as babies. Visualization develops when we are read to, which supports emergent reading skills later on.[10] This gives us all the more reason to unplug and snuggle up with a good book and someone you love.

In her inspiring book *See It. Say It. Do It!*, Dr. Lynn Hellerstein explores the concept of visualization against the backdrop of her experiences with her patients. Dr. Hellerstein, a leading behavioral optometrist, draws on her own extensive experience, both professional and personal, to share insights she gained about this powerful tool and how it can transform our development and help us realize our potential.

She discusses the numerous ways in which visualization can be defined, its deep-rooted history dating back to the days of antiquity, the science behind it, and the many ways it can help us successfully reach our goals. It is a tool for both children and adults alike and plays a role in four key areas of our lives that she has identified as academics, sports, social encounters, and personal growth.

One of the most fascinating aspects about her work is the model she created that can teach all of us how to develop our own visualization skills. She explains how to apply this in many different everyday situations through an extensive array of activities that can be done in a home or school setting. Insightfully, Dr. Hellerstein incorporates instructive exercises for proper breathing techniques that will greatly enhance the effects of the visualization techniques. In addition, she teaches that building awareness of body sensations is essential self-knowledge that directly influences one's visualization abilities and outcomes.[11] The power of this skill has been beautifully and artfully explored and articulated by Dr. Hellerstein in her book.

How successful we are at most anything is intricately interconnected with how we feel. Hunger, fatigue, weather-related discomfort, and emotional states all can affect our performance. In the case where there is an existing disorder in a dominant sensory system that is compromising our ability to perceive the world around us, we are at a big disadvantage.

When these disorders remain hidden and go untreated, the resulting effects can be heartbreaking. For children trying to grow and thrive in any learning environment, their senses must be fully engaged in order to keep up and succeed. If they are hobbling along with a deficient visual system, they will encounter considerable difficulty that will interfere with their progress and achievement. The consequences could follow them for life. Let's explore how this looks.

2

WHAT ARE VISION-RELATED LEARNING PROBLEMS?

You are reading this book with the hope of finding answers that might explain why a child in your life is struggling—your own daughter or son, your student, your grandchild. You may have searched, without success, for information that will help you unlock the mystery behind why he or she is travailing along and falling short of expectations and, worse, his or her own potential. It is painful to watch, and it is frustrating. It does not make any sense because you know this child is bright and capable and holds much promise.

Vision-related learning problems are not some newfangled, trendy class of ineptitudes concocted out of the need to relabel existing learning challenges that don't have any explanation. Often these get dubbed with terms that offer, at best, a vague representation of what is at hand. This is largely due to the fact that no one can actually explain *why* a child is struggling, despite extensive testing, observation, evaluation, and remediation.

These labels are general enough to evade accurate conclusions when, in actuality, none exist. At the same time, they are implicit enough to draw attention to the need for special services and, therefore, an unspecified yet unmistakable classification. The terms *perceptually impaired (PI)* and *neurologically impaired (NI)* are examples of these. What exactly the cause is that is impairing a child's perceptual abilities or brain function is not necessarily clear.[1]

Let's look at some revealing numbers. It is estimated that 25 percent of children in the United States struggle with learning problems. Now consider that 25 percent of all children have a vision problem that impedes learning.[2] According to the National Center for Health Statistics, 20 to 25 percent of children enter school with significant vision problems.[3] The greatest difficulty among learning-disabled children is with reading, affecting 75 percent of this population, and 80 percent of *these* children struggle with one or more visual skills.[4]

According to the American Public Health Association, "1 out of every 4 students has visual problems that are serious enough to impede learning."[5] Vision disorders are the fourth most common disability in the United States and the most prevalent handicapping condition affecting children.[6]

Sadly, these numbers are rising. The excessively demanding academic culture our children are now immersed in may actually be triggering learning problems and is a possible cause of this increase. We'll look at this more closely later on.

Undoubtedly it can be tricky to pinpoint the exact cause of a child's struggles. We know that a myriad of factors influence growth and development, which is why it is wise to consider the whole child when searching for answers. It is becoming more widely understood that difficulties may be rooted in physical causes, such as nutritional imbalances or allergies, as well as emotional disturbances or the presence of a developmental delay. Causes can be genetic, environmental, or social in nature.[7]

What too few people are aware of, however, is that a breakdown in the visual system can also be at the *core* of a learning disability.

These deficits directly affect learning, resulting in the classification of many, many children. They are also a health concern. Though the basis of a vision-related learning problem is functional, not medical, health comes into the picture as a secondary area of concern as increasing numbers of children are medicated due to symptoms that seem to interfere with their functioning in the classroom. This class of medications can have side effects that may interfere with appetite, sleep patterns, and mood, which can in turn affect overall health.

In either instance, many of the symptoms that a child exhibits may result in a diagnosis of a sensory processing disorder, dyslexia, AD/HD, or an executive functioning problem.[8] These problems may be managed with remediation in a special education program or with medication or both. However, a significant number of symptoms that are linked with some of these diagnoses are also present in a child who has a vision problem.

To fully grasp the reality of how the root cause of a child's struggles may be incorrectly diagnosed, consider that *fifteen out of the eighteen* symptoms linked with AD/HD are also associated with a vision disorder. *Thirteen out of the seventeen* symptoms of dyslexia can occur with a vision-based learning problem. When taken into account, then, that so few people know that vision-related learning problems exist, let alone how to evaluate for them, the potential for misdiagnosis is overwhelming.

Figures 2.1 and 2.2 categorically display the comparison of symptoms.

It is crucial to be aware that no matter how much intervention children get in the form of special education or medication, they will continue to struggle with learning unless their visual disorders are identified and corrected. In cases where there may be multiple disabilities playing out, the visual piece is so enormously influential that to disregard it will reduce the effectiveness of other therapies.

The problem is, awareness about vision-related learning problems is not universal. In their book, *A Parent's Guide to Special Education*, coauthors Linda Wilmhurst, PhD, and Alan W. Brue, PhD, educate parents as to how to traverse through the school system to get their child the help they need. One area they address is the Individualized Education Program (IEP). This program implements the coordination of a team of support services designed to specifically meet set goals and assessment procedures for a child who has been diagnosed with a learning disability.[9]

However, vision-related learning problems are not recognized as a disability because a staggering portion of our population does not know that they exist. Due to this, and the outdated means we rely on to examine children's vision, we are working within an educational model that is failing our children.

A 2012 study conducted by Ohio State University, with support from the Ohio Optometric Association, examined a group of 225 children with IEPs to ascertain the presence of vision problems. The team of researchers concluded that "there is considerable association between

SYMPTOMS OF DYSLEXIA
Compared to Symptoms of a Vision Disorder

SYMPTOMS	DYSLEXIA	VISION-BASED LEARNING PROBLEMS
Reversals	X	X
Letter confusion	X	X
Handwriting problems	X	X
Laterality confusion	X	X
Directionality confusion	X	X
Letter formation problems	X	X
Written language problems	X	X
Spelling difficulties	X	X
Problems with sequencing	X	X
Transposition, substitution, addition of words/letters	X	X
Poor short term memory	X	X
Poor word recall	X	X
Trouble learning sight vocabulary	X	X
Difficulty analyzing component sounds of words ("phonemic awareness")	X	
Difficulty with phonetic decoding	X	
Difficulty putting thoughts into words	X	
Trouble being on time or telling time and perceiving time	X	

Figure 2.1.   Symptoms of Dyslexia

Symptoms	AD/HD (DSM-V)*	Learning-Related Visual Problems (Kavner)	Normal Child Under 7 (Gesell)
Inattention *(At least 6 necessary)*: Often fails to give close attention to details or makes careless mistakes	X	X	
Often has difficulty sustaining attention in tasks or play activities	X	X	X
Often does not seem to listen when spoken to directly	X	X	
Often does not follow through on instructions and fails to finish schoolwork	X	X	X
Often has difficulty organizing tasks and activities	X	X	X
Often avoids, dislikes, or is reluctant to engage in tasks that require sustained mental effort	X	X	X
Often loses things necessary for tasks or activities	X	X	X
Is often easily distracted by extraneous stimuli	X	X	X
Is often forgetful in daily activities	X	X	
Hyperactivity and Impulsivity *(At least 6 necessary)*: Often fidgets with or taps hands or feet or squirms in seat	X	X	X
Often leaves seat in situations when remaining seated is expected	X	X	X
Often runs about or climbs in situations where it is inappropriate	X		X
Often unable to play or engage in leisure activities quietly	X		
Is often "on the go", acting as if "driven by a motor"	X		X
Often talks excessively	X	X	
Often blurts out an answer before a question has been completed	X	X	
Often has difficulty waiting his or her turn	X	X	X
Often interrupts or intrudes on others	X	X	X

Figure 2.2.   Attention-Deficit/Hyperactivity Disorder: Alternative Diagnoses

Copyright 1995 Patricia S. Lemer, M.Ed. All Rights Reserved—#B12
*DSM-V: *Diagnostic and Statistical Manual of Mental Disorders, 5th Edition*
Kavner, R. S. (1985). *Your Child's Vision.* New York: Simon and Schuster.
Gesell, A. (1943). *Infant and Child in the Culture of Today.* New York: Harper.

ocular anomalies and poor school performance. These problems are illustrated by the high prevalence of a variety of eye problems experienced in patients with IEP's."

They came away with another conclusion that they found shocking: "Out of the 179 that required treatment, 124 (69%) of the children with IEP's would have passed the school vision screening test. That is to say, nearly 70% of those children with an IEP were identified with treatable vision problems and yet would pass the vision screening because their vision problem did not affect their distance eyesight!"[10]

This is why it is so important for every child to receive a comprehensive vision examination prior to entering school and then yearly. To date, there are only a handful of states across the country that mandate these exams, among them Kentucky, Missouri, and Illinois.[11] Policies are a mixed bag nationwide. We lack a consistent method for examining children's vision that would ensure they receive the correct diagnosis.

It is also very important to understand that vision-related learning problems can affect every child, from those outwardly struggling the most to those who may be at the top of the class. Depending on the degree and number of deficits, as well as a child's inner resources, some kids may be able to compensate better than others. But the child who is getting all As and seems to be sailing along, who has a hidden visual disorder, may actually be working much harder than he or she would normally need to. How would you know then, you might be wondering, in a case where the child is seemingly successful? You can learn to look for the symptoms.

So what exactly do vision-related learning problems look like and how can we detect their symptoms? A child can have a deficit in one or more skill areas, and how these are expressed can vary greatly.

As defined by the American Optometric Association, learning-related vision problems are categorized into two areas: visual efficiency skills and visual information processing. Please note that the terms *learning-related vision problems* and *vision-related learning problems* are used interchangeably and have the same meaning. As with many things in life, it's about perspective. Those in the optometric community have structured the terminology around their focus, which is vision, whereas educators are learning centered, and the inverse of the term reflects this.

Visual efficiency includes the means by which the eyes physically take in information—through the systems of acuity, focus accommodation, vergence, and oculomotility. Deficits in any one or combination of these areas can make it difficult for a child to keep up with learning and can decrease the stamina needed to complete assignments and classroom tasks. This will impact the development of reading and comprehension skills, for starters.

Furthermore, children who are uncomfortable due to the physical symptoms from the stress their system is experiencing will instinctively take action to relieve this stress: they may look away from their work, wiggle and squirm while *in* their seat, find reasons to get *out* of their seat, and generally distract themselves. As we well know, these behaviors are not welcome to a teacher who is trying to maintain a status quo, and this will result in the child drawing negative attention or, worse, being *labeled*. This child is likely to then develop negative associations with learning and school, leading to increased behavioral problems or motivational issues. This scenario plays out far and wide in schools everywhere.

Visual information processing engages those functions in the brain that are of greater complexity. Within the extent of these processes, the spotlight is less on physiology and more on thinking and perceptual abilities that tie in with the other sensory systems in the body—vestibular, proprioceptive, auditory, and motor. These skills essentially allow for a person to make sense of what he or she is seeing and derive meaning from it. The importance of being adept with these processing skills cannot be underestimated.

Vision-related learning problems could manifest in many ways. There isn't any set modus operandi as to how they might present. There are, however, a whole host of signs and symptoms to be aware of that may clue us in to a potential problem. Knowing what to look for in the scope of a child's development would be a game changer. Certainly, this is where parents, teachers, doctors, and therapists play a key role.

Beyond the tests for acuity, through which eyeglasses or contact lenses would be prescribed if needed, comprehensively assessing a child's visual development would ensure that anything awry is caught and treated. Ideally this should happen early on, before it sets a downward spiral in motion. This needs to become the new gold standard. Such a proactive approach to detecting and treating these problems would alleviate undue stress and the likelihood of future struggle for children if deficits were discovered early enough.

When considering the possibility of the presence of one or more disorders, there are some tools that have been made easily available for parents and teachers to use. It must be noted that these are *not* for diagnostic purposes—only a behavioral or developmental optometrist is qualified to make a diagnosis. Rather, these are screening mechanisms that can alert us to the *possibility* of a visual deficit factoring in. They are designed to give us an indication of the likelihood that one or more disorders are present. Based on the criteria, one then comes away with a sense of whether further evaluation is warranted. If the results teeter on the border of "maybe," it is recommended to pursue looking into things further, given the huge ramifications if, in fact, a deficit does exist.[12] Screening tools are accessible on several websites listed in the back of this book, as well as in the appendix.

So what should you be looking for? Let's begin by exploring how one of the most common visual deficits plays out for a child.

Convergence insufficiency (CI) is a very common condition involving weaknesses in *oculomotility* and *binocularity*, resulting in the eyes being unable to work as a team. In normal binocular vision, both eyes coordinate to focus on one place, sending one image to the brain for interpretation. When CI is present, the eyes are focusing on two different places, consequently sending two images to the brain. This results in the child seeing double. Some of the symptoms of this condition include:

- headaches
- fatigue
- blurred vision
- eyes that feel sore
- frustration
- an inability to stay on task (sound like a familiar issue we hear a lot about?)

Now here's where it gets really interesting. As you now know, 80 percent of what we learn comes in to our brain through the visual system. When the brain has to make sense of seeing double, it tries to cope with this in one of two ways. The first line of attack is that it just clamors to make sense of two images. When this occurs, the percentage of information able to be processed in the brain is cut from 80 percent to a mere *50 percent*. That's a huge drop.

But fasten your seat belts for the second tactic the brain utilizes to try to cope—*it shuts down one eye*. The child doesn't know this or feel that he or she is only seeing out of one eye, but that's what is happening. When this occurs, the percentage of information able to be processed is cut to a dire *20 percent*. Imagine, then, the stress kids feel as they try to keep up in school. Moreover, coping with this condition is just plain exhausting.

When the eyes are not able to move steadily along a line of print due to the inability to automatically maneuver eye movements, tracking difficulties will occur. Precise motions enable us to move through a text, stopping long enough on a word to decode and grasp its meaning. Simultaneously, our peripheral vision is scoping out what lies ahead, preparing us to move forward and take in new information. It's a delicate dance composed of calibrated jumps and pauses that should flow effortlessly.

When the eye muscles are not able to control their movements accurately, however, the result is a loss of efficiency and slowed comprehension. Children will often lose their place or skip words and have to go back and reread the text because these interdependent vision systems are not coordinating properly to allow them to read smoothly. Fatigue and frustration set in.

Beyond convergence insufficiency, there is a multitude of other vision deficits that can impact a child. Here you will find explanations for all of them.

A child with *binocularity* or *oculomotility* problems may exhibit the following symptoms or behaviors:

- squints, closes, or covers one eye
- needs finger or straight edge to keep place when reading
- print blurs while reading
- complains of letters, symbols, or text bumping together, jumping, or moving while reading or writing
- omits letters, numbers, words, or phrases
- double vision

- loses place frequently when reading
- rereads or skips lines of text knowingly or unknowingly
- rereads or substitutes words when reading or copying
- writes uphill or downhill
- has a short attention span when reading, doing close-up work, or copying from the board
- misaligns numbers in columns when doing math problems
- poor handwriting
- tilts head while reading or writing
- excessive movement of head while reading
- poor fine or gross motor coordination
- burning, itching, or watery eyes
- headaches, nausea, or dizziness

Focusing problems cause an array of discomforts for children. Symptoms can occur in a child who needs corrective eyewear for a straightforward *acuity* problem. However, they can also occur in a child who has problems with *accommodation*, a deficiency that is less recognized. This skill allows us to quickly shift our focus from near to far distances smoothly. It also involves the ability to hold our focus for an extended length of time, as when we read.

In a classroom, this is a way of life. Children who cannot shift their focus efficiently will have a hard time keeping up in school, as they are required to move their eyes from the board to their desk, back and forth, frequently. When reading, they may not have the stamina to hold their focus. Children will intuitively seek relief by any number of means including putting their heads down on their desks, covering one eye, and avoiding close-up work.

Experiencing these discomforts may also result in behavior changes. Kids may frustrate easily, have a short attention span, lack motivation, struggle with copying from the board or their books, and fall short of working up to their potential. Symptoms and behaviors resulting from a focusing problem may include:

- eyestrain, headaches, and fatigue
- excessive blinking
- burning, itching, or watery eyes
- reduced comprehension

- slow reading and completion of work
- loses interest in reading
- holds book closely or positions face too close to desk for written work
- avoidance of near work
- short attention span
- daydreaming
- closes or covers one eye while reading or doing close-up work
- makes errors while copying during written work
- squints to see board; asks to sit closer to board
- tires easily
- rubs eyes after short time doing concentrated visual tasks

Kids who have difficulty with *visual motor integration* will present with more obvious physical symptoms reflecting challenges with coordination. When these problems exist, there is a faulty connection between information coming in through the eyes and the motor centers in the brain. Consequently, movement, coordination, and balance can be affected.

Children who struggle with *gross motor* issues will typically display problems navigating their way through space. They may have difficulty avoiding obstacles. Managing their bodily movements in relation to their body weight, the effects of gravity, and the task they are trying to accomplish, such as riding a bicycle or playing sports, is challenging for them. They may appear uncoordinated and clumsy or careless.

Fine motor issues play out with more dexterous tasks such as handwriting and activities that require deft, close-up hand-eye interaction. Children will have difficulty completing assignments on time due to the slow, lingering pace at which they work resulting from these challenges. And here again, frustration, the inability to stay on task, and falling short of potential are all outcomes of a child's strain and struggle.

Visual spatial skills, which are closely related to the visual motor integration realm, cause confusion in children who have deficits in this area. Being able to feel at home and comfortable in their own bodies and with their physical interactions in the world around them lays the foundation for the ability to recognize and understand relationships between tangible objects and abstract concepts.

For example, being able to orient oneself through the means of *laterality and directionality* also ties in with a fundamental understanding of the difference between left and right. This, in turn, is what enables a child to build on this developing awareness and ultimately see relationships between letters. In other words, knowing our left from our right is essential to knowing the difference between a "b" and a "d," "was" and "saw," and "36" and "63." Children with problems in these areas may display symptoms and behaviors that include:

- confusion between right and left, up and down, and front and back
- awkward pencil grip
- letter reversals when reading or writing
- difficulty with sequential tasks
- crooked, poorly spaced writing that may not stay on ruled lines
- misalignment of numbers when doing math problems
- more problems with written spelling than oral spelling
- may approach a line of text from either left or right
- paper overly rotated on desk when writing
- awkward posture when writing at desk
- a need to "feel" things in order to understand them
- presence of gross motor skill developmental delay
- problems with coordination and balance
- weak ball-playing and sports skills

Visual perceptual deficits include a broad category of ensuing problems and challenges for learners of all ages and abilities. While being cognizant of the notion that 75 to 90 percent of the learning that takes place in a classroom is processed through the visual system, we're left with a sense of how important it is for all systems to be operating correctly, how paramount this is for a child's success, and how huge a factor it is when something is not working right. Visual perceptual problems play out in numerous ways and are even more hidden and difficult to recognize unless you know that:

1. They exist
2. What to look for and how to uncover them

Children with a visual perceptual deficit may present with symptoms and behaviors that include:

- difficulty learning the alphabet
- difficulty remembering letters and numbers and writing them correctly
- letter reversals, omissions, and additions
- difficulty recognizing words
- confusing minor likeness and differences—run/ran; saw/was; on/one
- consistently confusing words with similar beginnings and endings
- may not recognize the same word if repeated later on the same page
- poor reading comprehension
- may read aloud softly to themselves to hear the text and compensate for lack of reading comprehension
- poor visual memory—slow to copy work due to need to frequently consult text
- difficulty concentrating
- difficulty understanding given instructions
- difficulty recognizing and remembering patterns
- easily distractible
- short attention span
- may be hyperactive or hypoactive

Visual figure ground deficits will make it difficult for a child to focus in on details while disregarding irrelevant surrounding information. Symptoms and behaviors include:

- concentrating on a specific word in a sentence or paragraph
- difficulty keeping their place when reading or doing math problems
- being easily distracted
- difficulty completing a letter or symbol when writing
- difficulty locating a specific object in a larger context, like a desk

Visual closure issues make it difficult to mentally complete visual information that is incomplete. Difficulties include:

- recognizing an object that is partially hidden
- visualizing missing parts of pictures
- mentally filling in missing parts of a poorly photocopied text

A *visual memory* weakness will make it difficult for a child to:

- remember the alphabet
- learn basic math facts
- read and spell words that are not spelled phonetically

Visual sequential memory deficits mean a child will be unable to correctly reprocess any symbol or sequence of symbols that the child has seen before. Difficulties include:

- general confusion
- poor ability to visualize
- long-term memory problems impeding comprehension

Visual form constancy problems are characterized by the inability to accurately understand an object as being the same despite changes in its position, direction, or orientation. This can cause children to feel uneasy about their ability to interpret the world around them. They may feel that they cannot rely on themselves to accurately understand information coming in. Difficulties may include:

- overall challenges with learning
- inability to recognize a letter, number, or symbol when it's presented differently
- inability to translate interpretation of a word between print and cursive[13]

The strength of these skill areas is, in some measure, dependent on the collective formative stages that a child progresses through in the scope of his or her development. Holistically speaking, we hope that our children are able to grow fully in every way throughout the span of childhood: physically, emotionally, cognitively, and socially. To be and *feel* healthy and whole, each of these spheres needs the chance to unfurl at the appropriate time.

When they do not and vision is affected, the process of vision therapy can help. Vision therapy (VT) consists of specially tailored activities that are implemented under the guidance of a behavioral optometrist and vision therapist. The activities help retrain the brain and eyes to function properly.

There is a beautiful, innate order to human development that has its own rhythm, timing, and logic. People are natural beings, and as in every realm of nature, our development and functioning are interwoven with all other manifestations within the greater order of the natural world. With the right conditions and support, humans have the capacity to course along and move through ages and stages quite ably. Of course, we know it is not always this simple. Physical environment, genetics, social milieu, relationship dynamics, economics, and a host of other factors influence how equipped we become.

In a conversation with Carol Kranowitz, author of the highly acclaimed *The Out-of-Sync Child*, she stated that observation plays an important role in the classroom. "Teachers, take note of a child who has any of these behaviors," she said, referring to the lists of signs and symptoms listed previously. "Many of these behaviors are observable to those of us even untrained in vision care."

Kranowitz shared a powerful story right out of her preschool classroom. She noticed that one of her students, a little boy, would always turn his head to the side when sitting in a circle for a group activity. All she saw was his profile. When she mentioned this to the boy's parents and asked them if they noticed it too, they responded that they had not.

Nevertheless they took him to be evaluated and learned that he was almost completely blind in his left eye. Treatment restored his vision, but they had caught it just in time. Had it progressed, he would have lost his vision in that eye permanently. There weren't any sophisticated diagnostics or assessments employed in the moments that led up to a life-altering course of action. A child's vision was saved and a difference was made purely because of the attuned senses and judiciousness of an attentive teacher.

In reflecting on her experience in the classroom, Kranowitz eloquently described the remarkable improvements she observed in her students who had undergone vision therapy: "When little kids received VT, it made them more confident, and it relaxed them so they could focus their energy on using their feet, singing, and clapping their hands. They were no longer hanging back; now I saw them fully engaged."

Teachers, never underestimate your own powers of observation and insight. It is often easy to feel overwhelmed by the endless demands and perpetual recycling of pedagogy, especially in this age of standards, testing, and canned curricula. The paperwork protocol alone is enough to max out your focus. But don't lose the trees through the forest. You read that right. As education has become a large-scale managed enterprise (the forest), we can easily lose the little people (our trees) in it.

Every once in a while, remind yourself why you've chosen to teach. Do whatever it takes to stay inspired and motivated because at the end of the day, when the bell rings at 3:00-ish, you are all that mattered to that child who spent the day with you. Your good sense, your attention, your intuitive prowess, and your know-how are what really matters to your student.

A benchmark met, an objective covered, or a test score—these are no match for the observable behaviors, actions, and signs that a child exhibits on your watch. You are now equipped with game-changing knowledge. This will only help you up your game, as one of the most influential adults in the life of a child.

Human beings are not born with all the vision skills we need. The abilities to use our eyes together as a team, focus efficiently, and move them fluidly are all skills that must be learned. In addition to these physiological abilities, the brain must learn how to use this visual information to understand the world.

- At *birth* babies cannot see clearly just yet, but in the first year of life their rapidly developing vision goes through important changes that lay the foundation on which their vision skills will be built as they progress through the toddler years and beyond.
- In the *first three months* of infancy, babies can only focus on objects up to eight to ten inches away. During this time, their eyes begin teaming and their vision starts to improve. They are able to track objects and reach for them as eye-hand coordination starts to develop.
- From around *five to eight months* of age, as eye movements continue to develop, the eyes now begin coordinating with the rest of the body. Depth perception, which is not present at birth, starts to

develop, and an infant now begins to see a three-dimensional view of the world around them. The development of crawling enables them to further coordinate their eyes with hand, foot, and body movements.

- Between *nine and twelve months*, babies are able to judge distance. Gross motor actions like pulling themselves up to a standing position, crawling, and trying to walk all help them improve coordination between their eyes and the rest of the body.
- By *one to two years* of age, the development of depth perception and eye-hand coordination should be well established. They are highly curious, interested in exploring the world with their senses, and able to use their vision to guide their hands as they grasp for objects and utilize them in productive ways, such as pointing and scribbling.[14]

Dr. Amiel Francke is a notable behavioral optometrist who maintains that the health of the visual system is linked to the systemic functioning of the rest of the body. He is known for believing in the principle that "the body and eyes are one."[15] Gross motor movement is vitally necessary for good vision development. Visual, sensory, perceptual, and motor skills interact in a mutually dependent relationship set in motion by innate blueprints drafted in utero.[16]

In their book, *Growing an In-Sync Child*, coauthors Carol Kranowitz and Joye Newman enlighten readers with information that teaches the importance of engaging children in a steady diet of sensory-rich activities so they can develop fully and grow to be "in sync" with their bodies, their psyches, and the world around them. What's more, they explain the profound role that vision plays in helping a child become "in sync" and the role that movement plays in relation to the child's vision development. Early on, visual skills grow through stimulation of the vestibular, proprioceptive, and tactile systems, along with perceptual motor skills, *as long as the child continues to move*, they emphasize.

"I believe that feeling good in your body makes everything easier. In order to feel good in your body, certain things have to have taken place in order for this to occur," explains Newman. "When Dr. Amiel Francke and I work together, sometimes he would send kids to me to work with them on the motor piece first, which they needed before they could handle the visual work. He felt they would need to develop a little more control over their body. And sometimes, I would send kids who came to me, to first see Dr. Francke to work with them on their vision. Since what I do involves how you move through space, when doing so you have to be able to perceive the space accurately."

Newman is passionate when she talks about the importance of movement to overall development and especially to vision. "Movement should be part of life, but the way we live today seems to inhibit movement. We prefer to play sports on screens instead of on actual fields. We are in awe of gadgets that do amazing things at the press of a button, but an equal or greater appreciation for the amazing things our bodies can do seems absent from our consciousness. Our bodies are the real tools for living, but when we replace the activity of our own natural inborn devices with the use of synthetic devices, we reduce our coordination, dexterity, and sense-ability. This is not healthy," she emphasizes.

"The way the world is developing now is fostering a lot of problems we're seeing in children," she adds. "We are going to see a lot more people wearing eyeglasses. The fact that babies are born with 20/200 eyesight is significant. They were meant to see at far distances. It's not until age seven that children are ready to do the close-up focusing required for reading and writing. There is variation with timing here, but by sixth grade, skills have fallen into place and proficiency evens out."

"Did you know that a normal child under age 7, at times, has most of the symptoms that are part of an AD/HD diagnosis?" writes Dr. Stan Appelbaum in his book *Eye Power*.[17] Check out the chart a few pages back and you'll see this listed. We seem to think there is something wrong with our children for exhibiting what is entirely normal behavior, and we are medicating them for this. In actuality there is something wrong with us for imposing inappropriate expectations on children, then holding them accountable when they don't perform up to our skewed standards.

In Finland, children do not begin attending school until they are seven years old. Interestingly, most of them do so ready and equipped with skills in reading and math. News of this is becoming common knowledge in our own country, as we've begun to examine other learning models in addressing the many growing concerns about our own. Yes, in Finland children have a much different experience going to school, resulting in what seem to be not only successful learners but also happier students.[18] Why is this?

There are a number of ingredients thought to contribute to the success of students and even education as a profession. Exceptionally high teacher standards are the norm. It is harder to get accepted into education programs than medical programs. While there are national content standards, teachers are trusted with the independence to design their curriculum around students' needs in order to meet them. Teaching as a profession is held in very high esteem. There are no standardized tests, and students aren't ranked.

What's more, those running the school systems through the government are educators, as opposed to politicians or business people. Play is highly valued, and children are legally entitled to fifteen minutes of free time every forty-five minutes. Overall, the environment in Finnish schools is one of collaboration, cooperation, and trust. Students spend more time outdoors and engage in critical thinking and problem solving in an atmosphere of discovery and learning for the sake of learning, versus getting good grades or test scores. In the early years, students learn how to learn through an emphasis on metacognition.[19]

Before you pack up and move to Finland (you were thinking about it, right?), we can embrace this as a teachable moment, while we survey the story of our own educational system unfolding as we speak. Yes, we are still writing it. We always have and we always will. However, we can no longer go about this with our eyes open but our minds closed to the guiding truth. We will help kids best by equipping ourselves with the unfailing knowledge about how they learn and grow through movement and sensory integration. Allowing for and *supporting* the natural order of development to take its due course in children is fundamental to success.

It is really about achieving balance. Standards by themselves are not a bad thing. It's when they are set out with inappropriate expectations that they can wreak havoc. "There's nothing wrong with standards, or goals, per se. It makes sense to establish a certain level of mastery for children to achieve, and to determine what students should be able to do and know over the course of a particular period of time—a school year, for example," writes education consultant and author Rae Pica. "But the standards should be realistic. It should be possible for the majority of students to achieve them, each at her or his own pace. That means the standards must also be developmentally appropriate and based on the principles of child development—designed with actual children in mind."

In a glaring contradiction to this logic, Pica points out that there are a combined total of *ninety* reading and math standards for kindergarteners under the new Common Core. All kindergarteners are expected to read according to these standards. She also reveals that of the 135 committee members who wrote and reviewed the Common Core Standards for K–3, not one of them was a K–3 educator or professional with expertise in early childhood development. [20]

Pica infers that there seems to be the perception among those writing the standards that children are smarter today than they used to be. In response to this assertion, Dr. Marcy Guddemi, executive director of the Gesell Institute, shares that "children are not reaching their developmental milestones any sooner than they did in 1925, when Arnold Gesell first did his research."

Is it that, perhaps, our sophistication as a civilization has produced a flawed perception of how we are to evolve? Has our fascination with our own ability to manipulate our environment led us to believe we can make ourselves smarter and faster if we just demand more, and do so sooner?

In a 2009 report by the Alliance for Childhood titled *Crisis in Kindergarten—Why Children Need to Play in School*, Edward Miller and Joan Almon advocate for reducing the two to three hours spent on formal math and literacy instruction (twenty to thirty minutes of which is test prep) and increasing time to engage in play and experiential learning. "Developmentally inappropriate practices are putting young children's health and academic progress at risk. It is time for a change," they uphold. [21]

Everyone who concerns themselves with anything related to children needs to understand the impact of what we are requiring of them. This includes the full spectrum of team members from parents, teachers, therapists, and pediatricians to those who mandate educational policy and design curricula and assessments.

For instance, Newman asserts that we should all know about visual fields. Don't feel bad if you don't. This is more than likely news to many of us. Right here and now, though, you are about to expand your knowledge base and come away feeling all the wiser for it. So what are they?

"Everyone has two visual fields," she explains. "Each eye has two fields. Anything you see that is to the right of your midline is in your right visual field. Anything you see that is to the left of your midline is in your left visual field."

Why is this practical know-how?

"Ninety-eight percent of us have the language system in our left hemisphere," she explains. "Anything that comes in to the right visual field goes to the left hemisphere where the language center is and is translated into language. Anything that goes into the left visual field goes into the right hemisphere and has to go thru the corpus callosum in the brain and be reversed so it can be processed in the language center."

"When we read to children, we do what's easier for us without realizing it, which is to put them on our right so that we're seeing things comfortably in our right visual field. What this means, though, is that they're seeing the text in their left visual field, which means we're making it harder for them," she elucidates.

Technology can also hinder the progression of vision development. Daniel R. Anderson, a psychologist at the University of Massachusetts, Amherst, focuses his research on television's impact on child development. In a July 2005 article written by Maggie Jackson for the *Boston Globe*, he was quoted as saying, "The evidence so far is that any hour they spend engaged in real-life activities is an hour in which they are able to learn much more, relevant to healthy development."

His research showed, for example, that children didn't learn a task as well from a screen as they did from a person in real life. Toddlers needed to watch a video showing how to remove a mitten six times before they were able to do it themselves. They only needed to be shown once by a real person in real space in order to get it. He does not see television as a useful tool for learning. In this article, it was also reported that only 6 percent of parents with children under two did not know that the American Academy of Pediatrics had come out with a statement recommending that no child should view any TV before the age of two.[22]

Dr. Leonard Press points out that the plasticity and malleability of the brain is very high even until the age of six. A leading behavioral optometrist who lectures internationally and is considered one of the pioneering doctors in the field, Dr. Press concurs with the belief that children should not be exposed to television before the age of two years. He has witnessed how kids become transfixed when staring at a screen, to the extent that they tune everything else out.

"When 3D entertainment displays came on the market, the manufacturers informed the general public about exercising caution in allowing children under the age of two to engage with them. This was a proactive, cautious move on the part of the entertainment industry, and one that deserves merit. The rationale was that we simply do not know what the effects are on the visual system in such young children, and playing it safe is the right thing to do. Whereas there aren't studies that conclusively show harm, the developing visual system is so susceptible that immersion at such a young age in an environment that requires such sustained focus might not be healthy. Until more studies are done as a lot of this technology is emerging, it makes sense to at least raise the possibility. Since we know video games for kids can be near-addictive, let's be cautious," Dr. Press explains.

This drives home the need for an environment that supports all of these processes during the delicate, critical, and dynamic early years of a child's life. When conditions are less than ideal, whether at home, at day care, or in school, the underpinnings of a deficit may become established. Hopefully this book will bring to light the need for understanding the importance of nurturing healthy vision development from birth.

We tend to take notice typically when children are older. Reliance on their visual skills becomes more concentrated and glaringly more obvious as they use their eyes more intensely as print gets smaller and paragraphs get bigger. However, the prerequisites for optimal vision that seem subtle must be recognized and given appropriate attention early on, to give every child the best chance for success.

With full regard to vision, a subject of lesser attention yet increasing importance must be mentioned here—concussions. As certainly as subtle imbalances can affect a child's visual development, physical injury to the head can induce problems instantaneously. Concussions are a form of mild traumatic brain injury. It is possible for traumatic brain injuries (TBIs) to cause vision-related learning problems to manifest as a result of injury.

Concussions are defined as "any transient neurologic dysfunction resulting from a biomechanical force."[23] This force causes the brain to move beyond the surrounding cerebral spinal fluid, which acts as a

cushion, and bump up against the inside of the skull. This causes bruis-
ing on the brain, what we call a concussion.

Symptoms may include:

- confusion
- headache
- dizziness
- vomiting and/or nausea
- blurred or double vision
- disorientation
- light sensitivity
- unsteadiness
- difficulty concentrating
- post-traumatic amnesia

Symptoms may appear immediately or can occur within the first
seven to ten days after the injury. They can take anywhere from up to
three months to a year to go away. In some cases, symptoms may persist
for more than a year. When symptoms last for more than three months,
a person is considered to have "post-concussion syndrome."

Concussions, whether mild or severe, can disrupt the normal neurological wiring in the brain. Since the visual system is incorporated
throughout so much brain terrain, there is the likelihood that visual
processing could be affected. Recent research has shown that more that
50 percent of those who have sustained a concussion also have visual
disturbances that may include convergence, accommodative, or eye
movement disorders. These symptoms can cause headaches and
blurred vision and may result in a decrease in reading speed and comprehension. A change in eyeglass prescription may be necessary in
some cases.

Symptoms can linger through the post-concussion syndrome. The
good news is vision therapy can help, and in most cases patients make a
full recovery. *It is extremely important to allow the brain time to heal.* A
behavioral optometrist should be included as part of the team caring for
the patient during the recovery process.[24]

"When a child has a concussion," Dr. Press notes, "vision is typically
the last concern on the list of symptoms and outcomes needing to be
addressed. It's simply not recognized as the important piece that it is in

the overall scheme of things. As children participate in organized sports at younger and younger ages, the incidence of concussions is becoming more prevalent. Here is an area where vision is a clear concern from both a health standpoint and an educational one. Teachers need to be aware of how concussion symptoms can impact a child in the classroom."

This is true for parents as well, so they may monitor their child's workload to ensure that it doesn't cause additional stress to an already compromised system that needs to heal. This could delay the healing process or cause the child to have setbacks. Ideally, parents and teachers should be on the same page with how to manage the child's school requirements. Temporary modifications might be needed until the child is fully recovered.

The story of Beth illustrates the importance of this. After her son was diagnosed with a mild concussion due to an accident that occurred during a game in gym class, the doctor told her he could return to school the next day. She was shocked to hear this since he had blurred vision and dizziness as a result of the injury, not to mention a whopper headache. She seriously questioned how he could function in school this way and decided to follow her own instincts and keep him home until he felt better.

The blurred vision and dizziness resolved considerably by the next day, but he still had a headache and was very, very tired. She continued to monitor his symptoms closely and followed his lead with regard to what he felt ready for. As it turned out, he wasn't ready to return to school for almost a week and a half, the same length of time that his headache lingered.

When he did go back, he was wiped out by lunchtime. So he continued on a moderated schedule of mornings only, until he could handle a full day. Certain activities, like looking at a Smart Board and writing at his desk, induced discomfort and brought back symptoms that had improved. Not knowing what to make of this, or how to manage his symptoms and recovery, Beth began looking for more answers. After consulting with several specialists, she reached out to Dr. Barry Tannen, a behavioral optometrist, for guidance.

Dr. Tannen gave Beth a different perspective that provided her with a sense of direction going forward. Dr. Tannen explained how her son's behavior and symptoms were the best indicators of the lingering effects of the concussion. He emphasized the importance of monitoring both his behavior and symptoms and explained how to do this. This, he reassured her, would be the best way to gauge what his activity level should be.

Dr. Tannen also described how the injury could make processing information difficult due to the strain on the sensory systems. He suggested strategies for minimizing stimuli, so these systems would not be overloaded.

Since the visual system occupies so much territory in the brain, a concussion can easily impact vision, which can factor into symptoms afterward. Making sure to reduce visual stimuli is especially important during the recovery process. Following up with a behavioral optometrist is recommended since they assess for the kinds of sensory processing issues that could result from a brain injury.

Beth's experience with handling her child's concussion coincided with the increase in attention the subject of concussions was beginning to receive in the media in late 2010. On the heels of her inquiries, there were articles surfacing left and right. It seemed everyone was catching on to the importance of closely monitoring children after a head injury. Of significance was the realization that often we are blind to what children are experiencing post-concussion.

On the surface, they may appear normal. Behind the scenes, however, in their brain, they may be dealing with a compromised sensory system that can cause all sorts of challenges. The insidious nature of the symptoms can make it difficult to pick up on what might be going on. In fact, they can be so subtle we might miss them entirely. This further supports the need for teaching child health-care and educational professionals about the effects of a brain injury on a child's ability to fully function.

An exciting new development in the effort to evaluate for possible concussions involves a test that can be administered directly on-site to athletes where head trauma is suspected. Mayo Clinic researchers have validated the use of the King-Devick test to assess for concussion symptoms in athletes, whether they play high school, college, or professional sports. The test is affordable, can be administered by nonmedical personnel, and delivers rapid, accurate findings.

It achieves this through measuring visual performance that requires saccadic eye movements, accommodative skills, and near vision reading of single-digit numbers displayed on cards. A baseline test is administered to athletes at the start of their participation in their chosen sport. If they are injured, the results of the test given at the time of injury are compared to their baseline score. If the time needed to complete the test is longer than their baseline, they are to be removed from play and evaluated further. It is especially useful in that it can detect concussions in athletes who may have had a silent concussion or who have not reported a brain injury.[25]

In light of the many ways vision impacts our lives and our lives impact our vision, appreciating its worth can give us a whole new perspective on its contribution to our quality of life, achievements, and degree of fulfillment. Exploring the bigger picture will help us take this appreciation to the next level.

3

"WHY HAVEN'T I HEARD ABOUT THIS BEFORE?"

Given that vision-based learning problems are so common that they affect one in four children, *why don't we know about them?* Two rationales will help shed some light on this.

The first explanation is that vision problems are inherently difficult to recognize given that they are most often hidden. When a child exhibits a speech problem, we can hear it. We have no way of knowing, however, what the world looks like to a child, and children typically don't question what they are seeing. It is highly unusual for a child to articulate how he or she sees, let alone describe any symptoms that may offer clues about why the child is having such a hard time in school. When they do, however, it can be dramatically revealing. These next few stories will illustrate that, in fact, it can be downright groundbreaking.

Janie's second-grade class was working on an enrichment assignment. The enrichment teacher was circulating around the room observing the students doing the activity. As she passed by Janie's desk, she saw her erasing frantically. There were dark smudges and holes in the paper where she had worn through from erasing so much.

Janie stopped, heaved a heavy sigh, and looked up at her. "You know," she said, "it's like magic. I write the lines on my paper, and then they move all by themselves and I have to start all over again."

This comment stopped the teacher in her tracks, wide-eyed at what she had just been told. Something clicked, and she knew what was going on. She relayed the story to the classroom teacher, who gasped and said, "Oh, my gosh! This explains it! For two years we've been trying to figure out what is going on with Janie, but no one can get to the bottom of it. She can't copy anything correctly off the board, and she is struggling so much."

She was familiar with vision-related learning problems and understood how incredible it was that in that moment they had experienced a revelation. Janie had actually articulated clues to a hidden vision problem at the young age of seven. This was extraordinary.

Another remarkable experience actually took place on a college campus, far and away from the formative primary grades. A class of graduate students at Rutgers University, who were studying to be guidance counselors, attended a lecture about vision-related learning problems. At the end of the presentation, the instructor did an exercise that allowed them to experience how it feels for a child who has convergence insufficiency to read, where everything looks double.

Two transparencies with the same text on each were positioned on an overhead projector so they were slightly misaligned and the letters appeared double. The students were then asked to read the passage. While they were trying to read it, the instructor moved the transparencies around a little, since a text may also appear to be moving to a child with CI. Of course, there were lots of moans and groans and a few gasps, which was the point of the exercise.

Later, after the workshop was over, a student named Risa approached the instructor and asked if she could chat for a moment. Risa then proceeded to declare that she didn't understand how she made it to graduate school.

"*That's* how I *see!*" she exclaimed, pointing to the screen with the doubled text. "And I didn't know until ten minutes ago that this isn't the way the rest of the world sees!"

Risa's professor stood there riveted to the floor, astonished at what she had just heard. Her mouth dropped open, and a look of disbelief washed over her face. She replied, as if in slow motion, "But you're one of my top students!"

Risa had a 4.0 GPA. This was testimony to how hard she has worked all her life despite a tremendous challenge. She spoke further. Her mother had always advocated for her, getting her the support she needed to help her succeed. Not all kids are so fortunate. Risa's life was changed that night.

These two experiences portray vision-related learning problems unfolding in a very young child and in a much older student who had plodded all through school with them. How might things play out for a student literally in the middle of his education?

Jonah, a sixth grader, brought home his report card and handed it over to his parents after dinner one night. It was a beautiful report card. They congratulated him on all his hard work and effort and showered him with praise. Jonah was a good student, and they were happy to see him continuing on his successful path into his middle school years.

His facial expression and body language, however, did not reflect a child who felt a sense of accomplishment, and it came as a surprise to them to hear what he had to say next.

"I just don't feel like I'm doing as well as this says I am," he said. When asked why, he said he felt like he was working harder than he should have to and just didn't feel like he was actually doing as well as everyone seemed to think he was doing.

Jonah's parents were familiar with vision-related learning problems and, after hearing this, took him for a comprehensive vision evaluation. Sure enough, and to everyone's surprise, they learned he was dealing with convergence insufficiency and several other vision disorders. Jonah went through four months of vision therapy and was completely rehabilitated, and his school-related stress went away as quietly as it came. His confidence was back on track, as was his comfort level with the demands of school. His parents were relieved, grateful, and delighted to see him return to himself again.

The concealed nature of a whole category of vision problems that many people are unaware of, and an incomplete understanding of what vision is, give rise to substantial limitations.

The second reason this subject is not widely known about is the lack of readily available mechanisms with which to educate others. Friend, you are wrapping your hands around a now widely available serious mechanism, so that this knowledge and awareness can belong to everyone, everywhere.

Behavioral optometry has evolved appreciably over the past fifty years. The field had its beginnings in the theories of Dr. A. M. Skeffington, who is considered to be the father of behavioral optometry. In the

1920s, Dr. Skeffington's visionary influence began to take hold. He had the insight to understand that other disciplines played a role in visual performance and needed to be considered when evaluating visual functioning.

At that time in history, he also had the foresight to recognize how near-point demands were taking their toll on the visual system and causing problems due to biological stress. He purported that human beings were not designed nor suited for these "culturally imposed near work demands." That was almost a century ago. Imagine what he would say today about our constant connection to screens and the high-pressure, test-driven academic culture that our children are helplessly caught up in.

Another pioneering thinker was Darell B. Harmon, PhD, an educator and kinesiologist. A fascinating field, kinesiology is the study of the mechanics and anatomy of the human body and how they relate to movement and behavior. His research findings brought to light concerns about the effects that the traditional classroom design has on vision and orientation in space.

Specifically, he drew attention to the issues of glare and contrast and the impact of classroom furniture design on posture. He saw a link between posture and visual outcomes, noting that when children struggle to feel comfortable in their seat, good posture can be compromised and poor body positioning can affect how accurately the brain processes visual input.

Dr. Harmon's insight into the importance of designing a physical classroom environment that would support optimal learning conditions promoted a greater understanding of the relationship between space, movement, posture, and vision. His work had a profound influence on the efforts of Dr. Skeffington and broadened the role of optometry as it sought to define vision development.

Dr. Nathan Flax, a well-respected behavioral optometrist whose highly regarded contributions are considered formative in the field, presented an insightful perspective about the development of reading skills. He drew a distinction between the visual skills that are needed for reading progress in the early grades and those necessary in the upper grades.

His analysis revealed that "in the early grades, 'learning to read' is dependent on adequate visual form perception and visual memory skills, which allow appropriate letter discrimination and sight recognition for words. In the later grades, once one has learned the rudiments of reading, efficiency of 'reading to learn' is related to efficiency of eye movement, accommodative, and binocular eye coordination skills." It is an inherently maturational process composed of cognitive, physiological, and neurological processes that are magnificently interdependent.

As the field of behavioral optometry evolved, it identified itself as a profession that correlated its practice and purpose with the function of learning. Dr. Skeffington's lectures and writings in the 1930s and 1940s identified the relationship between vision problems, reading, and learning. Collaborative studies with psychologists and special education teachers generated programs geared for struggling students that integrated this new knowledge.

As optometrists became more aware of the relationship between visual function and learning, the use of lenses and vision training began to increase. Professional archives expanded with ever increasing numbers of papers and monthly newsletter chapters documenting research findings, case studies, and clinical outcomes. The field was taking off as this knowledge revealed more and more discovery and insight into the role that vision plays in learning.

As new areas of visual dysfunction were identified, evaluative measures and treatment methods advanced. Families and schools began contributing to the process as optometrists reached out and asked them to share specific information about learning difficulties that proved valuable in assessing an individual's needs and formulating treatment options. Knowledge of the interaction between specific visual skills and learning practices unfolded to new levels of awareness. Research findings in the earlier part of the century provided the foundation on which new discoveries and procedures were shaped, paving the path for a world of opportunity to unfold with the potential to remediate concealed disabilities that would have otherwise gone unrecognized and untreated. [1]

The Gesell Institute of Child Development in New Haven, Connecticut, generated research-based observation and study of the role that vision plays in motor performance and behavior. The results of this work showed that vision is much more than a sensory action that merely records images, akin to a camera. Rather, these observations led to a greater understanding of the link between vision and problem-solving ability, as well as overall development. These advances added momentum to the expanding role of evaluation and therapy in helping children with vision deficits.

Behavioral optometry is a vital, growing field that continues to improve the lives of many people, children and adults alike, who seek to reach their full potential through treatment for visual deficits both subtle and striking. What's more, it has its work cut out for it.

In addition to the intrinsic presence of visual deficits needing attention, the profession is endeavoring to meet a growing need for intervention due to our cultural dependence on screens. Whereas this became apparent with the inception of video games in the 1980s and was drawing attention then, today's plugged-in lifestyle that requires our eyes to focus for unprecedented stretches of time on a fixed distance is enormously problematic. Behavioral optometry is seeing new trends in visual symptoms that were not present before.[2]

The National PTA is aware of the prevalence of vision-related learning problems, the success rate of treatment, and the overwhelmingly positive changes that occur for a child. At the 1999 National PTA convention, the following resolution was adopted unanimously:

Resolution
Learning Related Vision Problems—Education
and Evaluation

Whereas, It is estimated that more than 10 million children (ages 0 to 19) suffer from vision problems; and

Whereas, Many visual skills are necessary for successful learning in the modern classroom; and skill deficiencies may contribute to poor academic performance; and

Whereas, Typical "vision" evaluations/screenings only test for a few of the necessary learning related visual skills (distance acuity, i.e. 20/20 eyesight, stereo vision, and muscle balance), leaving most visual skill deficiencies undiagnosed; and

Whereas, Learning related vision problems, when accurately diagnosed, can be treated successfully and permanently; and

Whereas, Knowledge regarding the relationship between poorly developed visual skills and poor academic performance is not widely held among students, parents, teachers, administrators and public health officials; now therefore be it

Resolved, That National PTA, through its constituent organizations, provide information to educate members, educators, administrators, public health officials and the public at large about learning related visual problems and the need for more comprehensive visual skill tests in school vision screening programs performed by qualified and trained personnel; and be it further

Resolved, That National PTA, through its constituent organizations, urge schools to include in their vision screening programs tests for learning related visual skills necessary for success in the classroom.[3]

Dr. Leonard Press holds the conviction that a comprehensive understanding of what vision actually is must be established across disciplines. Furthermore, being informed of its role in development, learning, and behavior is critical. For all that vision is and does for us, its importance has remained in the shadows.

Katie Johnson, a teacher and author of the book *Red Flags for Elementary Teachers*, is a committed advocate. She has been teaming with local doctors to upgrade the vision screening policies in her state to include near-point evaluation. Currently, it only covers distance. Yet up close is where most schoolwork is done. It has been an uphill climb, but progress is happening slowly. She notes that this coverage so far only applies to first graders, but they intend to push for expansion up to third grade.

Johnson is committed to raising awareness about this for everyone in her home state. She points out that this has to be instituted on, ideally, a national level. In speaking to parent groups, she reveals that once eyes are opened to this, time and time again, people come forward and say, "You're talking about my kid."

"Working with the legislature has been a fascinating experience as well," she notes. "Every single time we communicate with them about this topic, including when we testify, one of two things happens. Every single person who learns about this says, 'Why aren't we doing this? Why haven't we been checking near vision?' The second thing that happens is at least one person speaks up and says, 'Yeah, I had a kid like that' or 'My niece/nephew/grandchild is like that.' And this is what gets people to get it—when it hits home."

Dr. Nancy Torgerson, a behavioral optometrist in Washington, holds monthly workshops in her office for parents, teachers, occupational therapists, physical therapists, and "anyone that loves your child," to teach them what vision is all about, complete with demonstrations and hands-on learning. Inevitably, someone usually speaks up and shares an experience that goes very far in revealing how vision problems can impact someone's life. This is both powerful and empowering.

Learning, and especially reading, are highly complex processes. It must be noted here that not every learning problem or reading difficulty will be rooted in a vision problem. It's not always a clear-cut path to finding solutions to these problems. In some cases, a child will need other remediation in addition to, or instead of, vision therapy.

"A medical doctor once told me that eye doctors need to be clear that vision is a *piece* of the whole puzzle. The doctor relayed that without making it clear up front that vision is a part of the whole picture, people get caught up in wondering about all the other areas that may be involved. Once I explain that I collaborate with many other professionals, and share the roles of those people, then the listener's internal questions are quieted and the person can hear what I am saying," she shares.

"Good vision does not guarantee good reading," explain Drs. Arthur Seiderman and Steven Marcus. "Some children whose vision therapy is successful may still need other forms of help—from a psychologist or a reading specialist, for example—in order to catch up in reading. This is especially likely if the child has had a relatively long period of failure before his therapy. When a child is profoundly discouraged about school and learning, the road back is not easy, and clearing away a visual obstacle is not all that must be done to rescue him."

It is possible to try vision therapy and find that it doesn't work because there is another underlying problem that is the cause of the struggle. VT is not a guarantee in every case. When vision is the cause, however, ignoring this will be detrimental. The positive impact that vision therapy can have on a child who is struggling because of a visual disorder simply cannot be measured. Its effects are all embracing and far-reaching.[4]

While we are highly dependent on our vision today, our way of life also places exceedingly great demands on this sense. The increasing rate of myopia (nearsightedness) is one result of this strain.[5] Then there are those that are less obvious, and here lies a possible additional explanation as to why so few people are aware of vision-related learning problems—we haven't quite caught up with ourselves. While we've forged ahead as a civilization and pushed our limits of intelligence, creativity, productivity, and innovation, we've fallen behind in understanding how we function.

"Considering our ratio of cones (5%) to rods (95%), it strikes me that we were not designed to sit for long hours engaged exclusively in foveal focus (close-up) activities, like reading, and watching TV or computer screens. The eyes need to actively experience the world as a whole for vision to develop fully," asserts Dr. Carla Hannaford in her book *Smart Moves*. Cones, which enable us to see color, and rods, which are highly sensitive to light, work in concert to give us the ability to see in two and three dimensions, during the day and at night, and peripherally as well as up close.[6]

We need to play some catch-up with respect to our understanding of our selves and our bodies in relation to our evolutionary trajectory. To move forward in a manner whereby we won't continue to compromise our ability to function as we seek to prosper and succeed, we will need to become conscious of how we operate visually. Fortunately, there are a lot of great resources that can help if you know where to look.

The Optometric Extension Program Foundation (OEPF) has grown to a membership of three thousand, runs several annual conferences and seminars that offer continuing education for practitioners, and publishes *The Journal of Behavioral Optometry*, a compilation of expertise, research, and educational resources. In addition, the OEPF creates materials to be distributed in eye doctor's offices for patient education. OEPF, then OEP, had its beginnings under the leadership of Dr. Skeffington, who served as education director for fifty years.

The College of Optometrists in Vision Development (COVD) provides a board certification process, qualifying practitioners as behavioral optometrists. Both OEPF and COVD are stellar organizations that promote awareness and education.

Listed in the References section in the back of this book are websites and books that will provide a wealth of information about vision, research, and practitioners. If you want to consult with a behavioral optometrist, you can find one in your geographical area through links on the websites.

With the right tools, we can all take on this mission. The good news is we have the tools. We just need to get these into the minds, hands, and hearts of every parent, teacher, and professional who cares for children. Together, then, we can all come to our senses.

4

"BUT I WAS TOLD THIS IS A BUNCH OF HOOEY!"

Each specialty in the professional eye care community has its own sphere of influence and each practitioner their own area of expertise that meets specific needs of their patients that they are expressly qualified to treat. There is plenty of need to keep everyone busy.

The differences between an optometrist and an ophthalmologist may seem subtle and deserve clarification. Whereas both types of doctors conduct thorough eye exams, an ophthalmologist is an MD and specializes in the anatomy of the eye, disease, eye health, and surgery. They do examine vision; however, they do so with a more anatomical application. Optometrists hold a degree of doctor of optometry, or OD, and also address eye health issues; however, their focus is more on the visual function of the eyes. Respectively, there are overlaps between these two specialties and ultimately each address eye health and vision since these functions are interrelated and interdependent.

The role of a behavioral optometrist is unique. In addition to their skills in general optometry, they have completed extensive continuing education that qualifies them to assess for, diagnose, and treat visual and perceptual problems. The Optometric Extension Program Foundation (OEPF), founded in 1928, provides more continuing education (CE) for the profession of optometry in this specialty on a yearly basis than does any other CE provider. The College of Optometrists in Vision Development (COVD) provides board certification for these specialists. [1]

Understanding the finer distinctions between areas of expertise is helpful when deciding which type of doctor to go to for any condition. Dr. Paul Harris, a behavioral optometrist who has contributed greatly to the field, offers a clever parallel and uses a computer analogy to explain.

"Ophthalmologists and optometrists come from two vantage points. The approach of ophthalmology is one that is far more hardware based, putting most attention to the physical structures of the eye and surrounding tissues. The optometrist's approach includes this but then looks far more at the software. The software is how we do the things we do with the visual system, and most of these skills are learned and developed," he explains.

You may have encountered opposing views if you've already explored this subject, or you may as you go on from here furthering your knowledge and speaking with others about it. There is, unfortunately, a lot of confusion out there, compounded with doubt. This is so important to tease out that this entire chapter is devoted to clearing up the uncertainty that sometimes dissuades people from seeking evaluation or treatment. Let's explore how this confusion is perpetuated. Hopefully by the end of this chapter, you will have perspective and clarity.

A parent who had learned about vision-related learning problems from her pediatrician took her son to a behavioral optometrist for an evaluation. The results showed that he in fact did need vision therapy, which she followed through on.

In addition to the activities that are done with a vision therapist, a child will sometimes need to work at home on activities to reinforce what is done in the office. Unfortunately, she did not follow through with the home regimen that was required for his vision therapy plan.

She didn't understand why VT didn't help her son and wanted answers. She sought out consultation with an educator familiar with vision therapy, who explained to her that her son didn't get good results because the home regimen was neglected, a critical component in the process. The mom shared honestly, to her credit, that in the follow-up conversation she had with her pediatrician after the vision therapy process ended, she did not relay the story in full to him. She did not tell him that they didn't follow through on the home regimen.

The pediatrician's takeaway, unfortunately, was that vision therapy doesn't work. He based his view on her account of their experience, which left out a crucial step in the process. The doctor didn't know the prescribed home regimen was neglected. He therefore formulated an opinion of vision therapy based on an incomplete and inaccurate portrayal of the process that was shared with him by his patient. Going forward, he will be skeptical of VT, and this may play out in any number of ways. However it plays out, his impression and subsequent message to others will be less than supportive.

Parents need to play an active role in the vision therapy process, to ensure that the exercises are being done correctly and especially to guide their children through the mental and physical challenges. VT is not easy, and parent participation also plays another very important role in the process—showing their child support, encouragement, and cheering them on when the going gets tough. Parents have an opportunity to help their child cross the finish line victorious, with newfound abilities and confidence.

When the VT process does not unfold in this way, however, a child's success will be limited. Parents come away saying that it didn't work or that it's quackery, and this feedback often makes its way back to whoever referred them. These inaccurate views based on accounts of incomplete treatment for these problems have challenged the efforts of many who are trying to help kids get the support they need.

If athletes want to achieve a high level of success, they train on a regular basis, not just once a week. As such, the eyes and the brain need regular reinforcement and practice to learn new patterns, and this can only be accomplished if there is fixed time set aside to do the exercises on a consistent basis. Vision therapy activities that are done at home usually take about fifteen minutes, though some developmental optometrists do not always prescribe home VT regimens. It depends on the doctor and the needs of the patient. However it's managed, its worth cannot be emphasized enough.

Some eye care professionals dispute the notion that learning problems can be vision based. There are a number of myths and, put simply, bad press out there about the subject. This inaccurate information gets out into the airwaves through examples like the one above and succeeds in turning people away or causing confusion, which doesn't help already stymied parents who want an answer to their child's struggles. These mixed messages may dissuade people from seeking evaluation or treatment. Why does this happen?

Miscommunication and misinformation are two of the biggest reasons there are controversy and confusion surrounding this field. The scenario above illustrates the effects of inaccuracy. Here's another example that brings to light what happens when disparity enters the equation.

A prevalent pamphlet on display in a pediatric ophthalmologist's office adamantly touts the message that learning problems are *not* vision based and anyone who is told otherwise is being seriously misled. The literature goes on to profess that these problems are in no way rooted in any dysfunction of the visual system and that no form of vision training would be beneficial. Furthermore, only a learning specialist would have the means to diagnose such problems and treat them accordingly. The overall tone of the brochure is absolute and depreciative.

Surprisingly, several years later, the same office begins to offer vision therapy. Yet alongside this service, additional incorrect and contradictory information about VT sits in its display that is endorsed and disseminated by major professional health-care organizations. That this all exists under the same roof alongside vision therapy services is both puzzling and disturbing.

Sadly, there are other causes behind the controversy. Believe it or not, politics has a strong influence on how this subject is understood—and misunderstood. One would think and hope that doctors would be immune to politics, since they are in the business of helping and healing. The unsettling reality is, however, that there can be competition among eye care professionals who hold to different models of vision care. This can actually hamper efforts to ultimately get everyone on the same page.

Like anything new, people who do hear about vision therapy will ask around to get second opinions and reviews from others. We are often skeptical of anything that claims to offer a solution, a cure, or a fix, with good reason. We have to be careful.

In the March 14, 2010, *New York Times Sunday Magazine* article, the unremitting controversy of this subject was probed in an article written by Judith Warner, author of *We've Got Issues: Children and Parents in the Age of Medication*. Besides explaining the role that vision therapy plays in helping kids who struggle, it explored the basis for disagreement and the claims that undermine its effectiveness.

Warner had done her homework well. In reaching out to the National Institute of Mental Health and the National Institutes of Health's National Center for Complementary and Alternative Medicine, she learned that no familiarity with this subject exists. The National Eye Institute is, however, familiar with the groundbreaking study showing that convergence insufficiency is successfully treated with in-office vision therapy. It's worth mentioning here that this study was, in fact, successful in turning the heads of critics and receiving a nod.[2]

This was a complex, multi-million dollar analysis that set out to prove that vision therapy is an effective treatment for this disorder. It was a randomized controlled study that did indeed prove the effectiveness of VT for this common condition. Dr. Mitchell Scheiman, the lead author and principal investigator of it, shares an interesting story that puts its impact and importance into perspective.

"A number of years ago researchers embarked on a study to prove that aspirin helps relieve a headache. For hundreds of years it has been common knowledge that aspirin is used to successfully treat this ailment. Nevertheless, the scientific community needed proof and so a study was mandated and carried out. It proved what we already knew," explains Dr. Scheiman.

Like the aspirin study, the convergence insufficiency study proved what doctors already knew for years. Yet it was felt that a formal study of this scope would bring validity to the subject and quiet the opinions of those who dispel its significance, which it did. The successful findings were publicized in both optometric and ophthalmologic journals and archives, as well as in a press release from the Mayo Clinic.[3]

The following news brief was published by the National Eye Institute, a branch of the National Institutes of Health: "The study concluded that office-based vision therapy in conjunction with daily exercises at home is the only effective treatment option for convergence insufficiency. Other treatment options—including home exercises called pencil pushups and computer software programs—were significantly less effective than office-based vision therapy."[4]

Vision-related learning problems have been recognized since the early 1900s, and effective treatments have been in existence since this time as well. Vision therapy is a multisensory process that engages the brain and the body. Since the other sensory systems are intertwined with the visual system, many therapy activities are designed to incorporate the use of the motor, auditory, and vestibular systems in conjunction with the visual system. Where faulty wiring in the brain can lead to inefficient visual processing and slowed progress, vision therapy can offer remediation.

Vision therapy, as explained by the American Optometric Association, is defined as follows:

> Vision therapy is a sequence of neurosensory and neuromuscular activities individually prescribed and monitored by the doctor to develop, rehabilitate and enhance visual skills and processing. The vision therapy program is based on the results of a comprehensive eye examination or consultation, and takes into consideration the results of standardized tests, the needs of the patient, and the patient's signs and symptoms. The use of lenses, prisms, filters, occluders, specialized instruments, and computer programs is an integral part of vision therapy. The length of the therapy program varies depending on the severity of the diagnosed conditions, typically ranging from several months to longer periods of time. Activities paralleling in-office techniques are typically taught to the patient to be practiced at home, thereby reinforcing the developing visual skills.[5]

Valid research on the merits of vision therapy dates back fifty-plus years. Documented studies over these past five decades have shown the effectiveness of vision therapy. There is an abundance of research backing this field that illuminates the scientific basis for the diagnosis and successful treatment of vision disorders.

The Effectiveness of Vision Therapy in Improving Visual Function, a lengthy report put out by the American Optometric Association, documented clinical research that lends significant support. The report cited more than two hundred references, and "the clinical research, scientific studies, and professional articles listed in the bibliography were first published in refereed scientific journals, meaning each were examined by outside experts before publication to validate their science, value, and research methodology."

As stated in the conclusion of this report,

> In response to the question, "How effective is vision therapy in remediating visual deficiencies?" it is evident from the research presented that there is sufficient scientific support for the efficacy of vision therapy in modifying and improving ocular motor, accommodative,

and binocular system disorders, as measured by standardized clinical and laboratory testing methods, in the majority of patients of all ages for whom it is properly undertaken and employed. The American Optometric Association affirms its long-standing position that vision therapy is an effective therapeutic modality in the treatment of many physiological and information processing dysfunctions of the vision system. It continues to support quality optometric care, education, and research and will cooperate with all professions dedicated to providing the highest quality of life in which vision plays such an important role.[6]

Long before formal vision therapy came about, exercise to promote eye and vision health had been intrinsic to thousand-year-old wellness disciplines. Yoga includes specific eye exercises in its practice, as does qigong (pronounced chee-gung).[7] Whereas yoga originates from India, qigong and its more familiar cousin, tai chi, originate from China.

Both disciplines are similar in that they are wholly integrated mind-body approaches to wellness. While considering all the systems of the body, both yoga and qigong pay special attention to the eyes. Each has specific movements designed to tone the eye muscles. Ancient health wisdom had the insight to know the value of this type of exercise.

The importance of visual hygiene is less on our radar today, an effect of modernization and becoming increasingly disconnected from our bodies and the natural world. In his book *Last Child in the Woods*, award-winning journalist Richard Louv discusses at length the cost of progress and technology to our inborn sensory abilities. "Public education in enamored of, even mesmerized by, what might be called silicon faith: a myopic focus on high technology as salvation," he writes. Fascinating that he uses the term *myopic* metaphorically.

Computers are incredible instruments and have their place in our world. They are here to stay. However, it is their usage that needs tweaking. "The problem with computers isn't computers—they're just tools; the problem is that overdependence on them displaces other sources of education, from the arts to nature," writes Louv. "As we pour our money and attention into educational electronics, we allow less fashionable but more effective tools to atrophy."

Recent research efforts are examining how computer use is affecting children's development, especially with regard to vision. The findings are showing detrimental outcomes, especially at a young age. We should be concerned about the long-term effects of this. Since this is playing out in real time, we won't actually know until sometime down the pike, compounding the uncertainty. [8]

The College of Optometrists in Vision Development cautions parents to avoid being misled by mass-marketed independent eye exercise programs that claim to strengthen eye muscles. It is important to understand that optometric vision therapy does not seek to strengthen eye muscles. Eye muscles are already very strong. Rather, its goal is to "improve the coordination and efficient functioning and processing of the visual system," as stated in the journal of the Australasian College of Behavioural Optometry. [9]

Dr. Leonard Press goes the distance to educate people about why vision therapy is the game changer that it is, providing a detailed FAQ link on his website that addresses in depth the origins of the misinformation and misconceptions about vision therapy. He shares insightful perspective with his patients.

"Unlike drug studies, in which the patient takes a placebo pill, it is challenging to design a placebo therapy group," he explains. "Placebo therapy must be designed well enough that neither the patient nor the therapist knows that the therapy is not directly addressing the condition. The CITT (Convergence Insufficiency Treatment Trial) group did a brilliant job designing this group, which is why they were able to generate such a good rate of improvement that came about from improving sustained visual attention—in fact a couple of percentage points greater than the home-based computerized therapy group!"

Dr. Press goes on to justify the significance of this study, bringing to light the challenges inherent to designing the types of research studies that hard-core research-loving scientists rely on to validate treatment. [10]

Let's explore this further. Consider this: If all other intervention has failed to help the overwhelming number of children who are struggling to overcome learning challenges and meet with success, but vision therapy helped them do so, what is the argument? Each and every individual case where a child has been declassified, has been taken off medication, has become a reader, has at last begun to thrive, or all of the above *because* of vision therapy should qualify as hard-core evidence. Appendix B is composed of testimonials from the parents and children who experienced this.

Patricia S. Lemer is a licensed counselor with more than forty years of experience diagnosing children with learning and behavioral issues. Author of *Outsmarting Autism* and the retired executive director of Developmental Delay Resources (DDR), which merged with Epidemic Answers in 2013 and for which she now serves as board chair, Lemer addresses the importance of being informed. She provides support for parents seeking to educate themselves with accurate and reliable sources in her article "Choosing an Eye Doctor," which is available on the DDR website listed in the References section in the back of this book. Equipped with extensive knowledge about the impact of vision on child development, she writes: "Scientific evidence indicates that interventions such as Vision Therapy, used by behavioral optometrists, work. If your child has developmental delays of any kind, choose to have all aspects of vision evaluated. The American Optometric Association publishes a monograph, The Efficacy of Optometric Vision Therapy, containing 238 references."[11]

In the medical journal *Transactions of the American Ophthalmological Society*, eye muscle surgeon and researcher David Guyton, MD, states: "We [ophthalmologists] have probably abdicated the study of accommodation and convergence to the optometric profession. A perusal of the literature will reveal that most of the advances in this area are being made in the optometric institutions by vision scientists who use definitions and terms with which we are not even familiar."[12]

Conceivably, some of the skepticism that exists may be a side effect of a lack of understanding.

Dr. Guyton, along with his colleague Dr. Michael Repka, both of whom are world-renowned ophthalmologists, describe how they're beginning to consider the connection between vision problems and reading ability, especially in low-income families. In the article "Classroom Insights," published in the 2014 annual report of the Wilmer Eye Institute at Johns Hopkins University, they discuss how they and their colleagues are examining whether the origins of a reading difficulty might be based in a visual problem. In collaboration with the Johns Hopkins School of Education, they have launched what is being referred to as a pioneering study to seek answers to these questions and solutions to these difficulties.

This exciting effort contains many ingredients that, when combined, can produce a potentially wonderful result. The ophthalmology researchers bring to the mix expertise in the realms of public health and clinical research and care. The education research is under the auspices of Robert Slavin, PhD, the director of the education school's Center for Research and Reform in Education. Their collective goal? Read on.

"This is really an epidemiological study and is pretty aggressive in its plan to identify, intervene and retest all within a single school year. If we're successful—and we have every reason to believe we will be—the next big step will be to create a system for schools to manage vision problems as a normal part of their reading program nationwide," Slavin says.

"You're talking about a lot of kids—millions, perhaps. It would have an enormous impact on real lives," David Friedman, director of the Dana Center for Preventive Ophthalmology, says.[13]

Music to the eyes, right? If we help these millions of children succeed, we will all prosper. In fact, we may be on the cusp of real transformation and cooperation.

The Interdisciplinary Council on Development and Learning (ICDL), in its *Clinical Practice Guidelines*, published a chapter titled "An Ophthalmologist's Approach to Visual Processing/Learning Differences," by Harold Paul Koller, MD. The purpose of the ICDL, founded by Dr. Stanley Greenspan, is to promote an interdisciplinary approach to meeting the comprehensive needs of the developing child, with the goal of helping each child reach his or her full potential. This ideology takes into account all of the factors in a child's life that directly affect the child's development, including vision.

Dr. Koller elucidates in eloquent and practical terms what must occur so that we can all be on the same page. Acknowledging that historically the ophthalmologist's role—their part in the whole—has not included an understanding of the interplay between visual function and academic success, he asserts that gaining this awareness is essential.

"This limited role for ophthalmologists in treating children with learning disorders is now being displaced by a move toward an interdisciplinary approach. The ophthalmologist is often the first expert to whom the pediatrician refers a child suspected of having a learning disorder. Educating ophthalmologists in the medical and non-medical conditions and situations that could affect learning in a child or older individual will help ensure that a patient receives appropriate, effective, and timely remedial treatment," he asserts.

To take this progressive view one step further, he adds, "It is important for one professional to take the responsibility of coordinating all the specialists actually involved in the care of any patient with a learning difference. It doesn't matter what that person's specialty is, so long as he or she is knowledgeable in the general field and has the motivation, passion, and resources necessary to coordinate the efforts of numerous physicians, psychologists, educators, and allied health professionals, such as occupational therapists, physical therapists, optometrists, and speech and language therapists."[14]

Thus he recognizes the need for cross-contextual awareness and understanding among all medical and developmental professionals who care for children. Furthermore, he makes the perceptive observation highlighting the need for coordination of care—a sensible ideal we should strive to meet.

As cited earlier in this chapter, Dr. Paul Harris strongly advocates for the need for dialogue between professions and assures us that this is occurring, though not often enough.

Robert Nurisio is a highly respected, distinguished vision therapist and model for his peers. In addition to treating patients with tremendous skill and compassion, he writes and advocates widely on this topic. Robert wrote "Myths and Realities . . ." which appeared in the blog *VT Works*, which he founded. An excerpt directed at unraveling the myths themselves is printed here. Robert writes:

> Let's inject some logical thought into some illogical assertions, with a goal of converting myth into reality.
> **Myth #1—Vision and Reading Are Unrelated**—As any normally sighted person who's attempted to read while blindfolded will attest, the task is next to impossible. If you can't put your eyes on it, you can't read it. Your eyes are your windows to the world, your vehicle for interpretation, your camera for photographing; and since our brains cannot absorb written ideas by osmosis, our pictures are necessary. Whether you buy the idea that vision plays a small or large role in reading, our blindfold experiment proves that vision has to exist in order for reading to occur. By virtue of the need of open eyes, we identify vision playing some role in reading, which for the moment establishes the relationship. Vision and reading are related.
> **Myth #2—If You Can See It, You Can Read It**—With the blindfold removed the picture reappears, guaranteeing reading abilities,

right? Wrong. Haec cogitatio est praemissa tot fabulas ad visionem (Latin for "this thought is the premise for so many myths related to vision"). The Latin is there plain as day for you to see and as clear as anything else on this page, but you cannot read it—unless by some fluke you read Latin fluently. The English words you understand are printed just as clearly as the Latin you couldn't; the main difference being interpretive skills. Your eyes took a picture of the English words and sent them to your brain for interpretation, and in turn, your brain offered them meaning. With the Latin words, no interpretation was available due to a lack of experience, but you can see the Latin words just fine. There is more to reading than just seeing clearly.

Myth #3—Reading Fluency Is Unrelated To Tracking Ability—As any Optometrist, Vision Therapist, astute Vision Therapy patient and even Ophthalmologist will testify, this one is actually part truth. Tracking, by definition, is the ability to constantly and continuously align the eyes on a moving target. Since very few elementary school students desire to, or are asked to, read their text while it is flying across the room, tracking becomes a secondary or even tertiary concern. Reading usually does not require anyone follow a moving target. Reading is truly based in saccadic ability (jumping from one point to the next—such as word to word) and fixation ability (steadying the eyes on a fixed target); the latter of which is neurologically linked to tracking, but requires zero movement. On a deeper level, the jumps from word to word (saccades) are controlled by a completely different neurological process than tracking. Apples and oranges.

Semantics can often be a matter of splitting hairs, and some may argue that is the case here. However, since we think and communicate in language, the choice of words becomes important in detecting the facts, and understanding the myths and realities. I believe the language used separates those who understand the truth from those who do not.

Myth #4—There Is No Research—When I was a boy, I believed the red cars went faster than the rest, based on absolutely nothing. Now some 30 years later through my own evolution, the thought makes me laugh, and the boyhood impression is something of the past. Thirty years ago there may not have been research on VT's efficacy, but now there is. Like the red cars, it's time to outgrow our old ideas, and replace them with more current facts, which are based in reality.

Myth # 5—Vision Therapy Doesn't Work—There will always be a faction of the population that believes this, the same as there will be groups believing Elvis is still alive, martians live in Area 51, and Neil Armstrong's televised landing on the moon was nothing more than an elaborate hoax. Anyone taking a serious look at Vision Therapy though will discover the logic, the premise, and the method behind it; further understanding that our eyes capture pictures of the world for our brain to process, and are an integral piece in our understanding of the world. If this were untrue, a blind person would have no problem reading the printed word, driving a car, or throwing a baseball around in the backyard. These tasks require an accurate visual picture in order to create an appropriate response, making them impossible to the blind—and challenging to those sighted folks who cannot accurately determine the where, the what and the why through their vision. Vision Therapy teaches us not only how to move our eyes more efficiently, but also how to understand what we see, and even what to look for.

If you're still not sold on the impacts of vision on learning and life, perhaps you can admit there is at least enough information available to research yourself, rather than just believing the naysayers because they say you should. Knowledge is power, and with the knowledge of what VT can really do, I believe I know the conclusion you will reach through your research. [15]

Pacific University School of Optometry, in Oregon, offers a progressive model of study for students entering the eye care profession. In addition to the opportunity to become an optometrist, two master's degree programs are offered to supplement future practitioners' qualifications and enable them to better serve the needs of patients.

A master of education with a concentration in visual function in learning bridges the worlds of optometry and education by teaching students about all components of the reading process and how these interrelate with vision. Cultivating a familiarity with learning processes will immeasurably benefit behavioral ODs as they treat children with vision-related learning problems.

Students also have the option to pursue a master of science in vision science. This degree prepares students for teaching or research in the ophthalmic field, concentrating on all aspects of vision that may be specific to either ophthalmology or optometry. What a great example for the entire eye care community! With this program we see a supportive, complementary effort that will serve to enhance each aspect of vision care in a cooperative paradigm.

This model program exemplifies how different branches of learning can come together for the greater good and realize that each of their respective specialties has a place in the world. The opening objective that is stated in the Hippocratic oath is to "first, do no harm."

While it is typical for pediatric ophthalmologists and developmental optometrists to not see eye to eye on much of anything, there are exceptions. Two extraordinary individuals have committed to building bridges between their respective professions.

Thomas Lenart, MD, PhD, doesn't fit the traditional pediatric ophthalmologist archetype. He is, one could say, "open minded" regarding patient care. Perhaps this characteristic was nurtured through life experiences that are different from what is encountered by most pediatric ophthalmologists. For instance, he spent two years as a Peace Corps volunteer in French West Africa. He also obtained a PhD prior to completing medical school.

When he bought his practice, the physician he bought it from had done research on the area of accommodation, an area that most pediatric ophthalmologists do not even test. His partner in the practice was an optometrist that understood the orthoptic benefits that tools such as flip lenses and Brock strings could bring to patients. Over time it was apparent to Dr. Lenart that there was more to vision therapy than what his partner was doing in the clinic.

Since his office had the policy of referring the "tough VT cases" to Dr. Nancy Torgerson, a behavioral optometrist, an established line of referral was in place. It just so happened that Dr. Torgerson had her own questions regarding many of the surgical management decisions and more traditional "ophthalmologist" approaches to pediatric eye care.

A mutual collaboration began. Once trust was established, questions began to flow back and forth. Dr. Lenart had observed a strong referral pattern from occupational, speech, and physical therapists with his partner and other developmental optometrists in the community. Dr. Lenart was curious as to what these therapists wanted from the exam/ evaluation that aided in helping the mutual patients. In discussion with Dr. Torgerson about this topic, Dr. Lenart recognized that what was being sought by the therapists was being delivered by the developmental optometrists and probably not by the pediatric ophthalmologists.

This sparked hundreds of questions about how visual function is more than 20/20; how one may see 20/20 but not know where one is in space; how toe walking could be a visual misinterpretation of space; how vision can impact reading; how vision can impact learning; how AD/HD is three times more likely in those with convergence insufficiency than in the general population; how smooth tracking of a target is not the same as the saccadic eye movement needed with reading; how problems hitting a baseball could be a function of the eyes not teaming together; how having the eyes cosmetically straight is not the same as having them work together; and how these functional visual skills could be developed in optometric vision therapy.

After more than five years of seeing this in action, Dr. Lenart and Dr. Torgerson decided to bring the collaboration into closer physical proximity, and opened a vision therapy satellite office in his building. This new satellite clinic was much more convenient for some patients who were traveling a distance to vision therapy sessions. The satellite office has not only secured a foothold as a progressive model, but it has grown since its beginnings in 2013.

The questions and discussions continue to this day, as Dr. Torgerson and Dr. Lenart still have much to learn about each other's perspectives. Notably, there is mutual respect, and each doctor wants to understand more from the other to be able to be their best for their patients. They speak on collaboration, as their dream is to have other ophthalmologists and optometrists work together to help patients get the care they need.

Ultimately, it is the decision of every individual seeking care. Innocent, dependent, vulnerable young human beings need compassionate, responsible, ethical grown-up human beings to help them grow up healthy. It's time to readily work alongside each other, on the same team, so we can make this happen. Every one of us has something to give.

5

SENSORY OVERLOAD

Plugged In, Overworked, and Overwhelmed

There is the saying that life goes by in the blink of an eye. If we could all just step off the treadmill of our routines for a moment and contemplate this well-worn idiom, we might have the breath to consider how quickly life passes us by and how much of the important stuff we might miss in our race to get to wherever it is we are going. How the world came to be this frenetic place is a question about which we could deliberate and gather many opinions and write a whole separate book about, but one may argue that our consumer-centric culture is the hub that our lives have evolved to revolve around.

What does this have to do with vision? More than meets the eye. Our children are bearing the brunt of our society's skewed priorities. Today's kids are exhausted, stressed, anxious, and feeling an unprecedented degree of pressure. As parents, many of us feel their pain. Ask a teacher, and that teacher will spew forth his or her frustration: too many standards and tests that snuff out a child's innate curiosity to learn about the world and a teacher's inborn passion to help the child do so; too many teachable moments lost to the demands of a canned curriculum; too many creative minds and hearts stifled by a system that swallows up potential and spits out mechanized products of force-fed information.

If our children are ever going to learn how to think for themselves, tap into their own talents, and become lifelong learners, there is much that needs to be revisited and revitalized in our educational sphere. Take note—it is not the sole responsibility, or fault, of teachers or administrators. School personnel are caught up in a larger cultural momentum. These challenges are part of something bigger.

While it is daunting, we can hone our focus on where to begin to understand this phenomenon if we muck through the overwhelming multitude of needs and begin with the basics: our children have the birthright to a healthy and safe childhood. Yet all too often their essential needs that would ensure this are sacrificed in the name of progress—and not just academic.

Many believe that behind all the standards, testing, and formalized core curricula is the root of all the pressure and demands—economic and material gain. We are quite possibly burning our children out before they reach college with the ultimate objective of turning out skilled workers who can compete in the world market. Culturally, we are driven by the need to remain number one.

How ironic this is on so many levels. All through childhood, and especially in school, we try to teach kids that being the first is not always what's important. After all, we can't be first in line all the time, and it doesn't even matter because we will all get where we are going anyway. Ask a kindergarten teacher how many times that's been said to students fearful that, if they weren't first in line, they would somehow get left behind!

Trying your best and being proud of your own personal achievements is what we all want our children to feel. But what earns the spotlight today is being on top. Unfortunately, conditions on the way to the top have come to include emotional and physical *un*wellness, social disconnectedness despite all the technology, and environmental degradation. These issues challenge us individually, and this is a microcosm of the stress, imbalance, and distorted value system that we are grappling with today on a global scale.

This is not to say that economic stability and prosperity are not worthy endeavors.

We want to be able to sustain our lives and live comfortably and feel contented. We must not strive for these reasonable goals, however, in ways that compromise and even destroy the ground beneath our feet or our ethics and sensibilities.

Dr. Joel Zaba, a behavioral optometrist in Virginia, shares his perspective. As society has grown ever more complex, he points out, and jobs require a greater sophistication of skills, literacy among adults is necessary both to keep up as workers and to keep us in the game. Lacking this, societies become compromised both economically and socially.[1]

There are some readily identifiable factors that are playing into the stress our kids are experiencing. One of them is homework. This is a controversial subject and has received, thankfully, a lot of attention in recent years. One of the reasons for this is that parents are beginning to speak up and challenge, thankfully, the increasing amounts of homework that children are getting in kindergarten (yes, really) right on up through high school.

The detrimental effects of this burden are numerous. The long hours spent sitting at a desk mean less time to run around and play, depriving children of much-needed exercise. Indeed, excessive homework may even be a contributing factor to obesity and other sedentary lifestyle health issues. Beyond this, we are learning that more sitting and less movement actually detracts from learning capacity.

In his book cited earlier, Richard Louv closely examines the losses incurred from the disappearance of unstructured, outdoor playtime where children have the chance to use their imaginations and explore their environment. Opportunities for this kind of play are being increasingly identified as a crucial facet in the healthy development of the whole child.

Ideally, our children need to be outdoors in nature and allow their bodies and imaginations to run free. For a myriad of reasons elucidated by Louv, opportunities for this have dwindled dramatically, and we are only beginning to understand the resultant effects. As sad as this is, our more programmed physical outlets in the form of recess and gym time are being cut back in favor of academics. This is a big mistake.

The research is piling up showing the positive effects that gross motor movement has on brain function at any age. Increasingly, these studies are confirming that children's cognitive abilities develop better when they engage in physical activity that stimulates multiple sensory areas in the brain. In his book *Teaching with the Brain in Mind*, Dr. Eric Jensen articulates why recess, physical education, and plain old play are important. One of the world's leading educational neuroscience researchers, he explains the mind-body connection through several contexts and offers suggestions for how to incorporate movement and play into school settings to develop cognition.

In the summary of his book, he writes, "Evidence from imaging sources, anatomical studies, and clinical data shows that moderate exercise enhances cognitive processing. It also increases the number of brain cells. Schools that do not implement a solid physical activity program are shortchanging student brains and their potential for academic performance. Movement activities should become as important as so-called 'bookwork.'"[2]

Brain Gym is a movement-based program founded in 1987 by Dr. Paul and Gail Dennison, a husband-and-wife team of educators. The history behind the research that inspired their pioneering work is fascinating, and you are hereby encouraged to check out their website. It's listed in the References section of this book. It is of great interest to note that Dr. Dennison collaborated with a developmental optometrist in the initial stages of his research that led to the creation of *Brain Gym*.[3]

Brain Gym employs kinesiology principles that have been shown to effectively foster improvements in cognition through movement. So effective and revolutionary, its program and philosophy are cited throughout much of the literature in this field, including the best-selling book *Smart Moves* by biologist and educator Dr. Carla Hannaford. Dr. Hannaford's work is also viewed as groundbreaking, and she eloquently weaves storytelling in with her research analysis to educate readers about the integration of mind and body.

In a remarkable and moving story, she describes her own learning curve as it unfolded over the course of a year while observing dramatic changes that occurred in a student who participated in informal movement and socialization experiences. Intrigued, her observations led to many questions and, ultimately, the work that culminated in her book. In essence, she discovered that "the body was just as important as the brain when it came to learning." This book is for all of us, as it innovatively examines the whole of human experience and how it all ties together to nourish our thinking, understanding, and creativity.[4]

Lamentably, with all the assignments that kids must juggle after a full day of school, there is little time left in their day for play. Drs. Jensen and Hannaford each make the case for seriously questioning how we educate our children and what our expectations and goals should be. We are fortunate to have in our midst these scholarly thinkers and investigators who are establishing justification for the moving of mountains. We are also fortunate to be sharing these ideas with each other through these pages.

It's going to take all of our collective brainpower and resolve to move these mountains. We need to spur a movement about movement so we can achieve movement! Game on.

Not only are children under a lot of stress from the amount of work they have to do at home, but families are also feeling high levels of stress and frustration because of the bite that homework takes out of precious family time. Family dinners, where much needed and deserved bonding time brings everyone together after a long and busy day, are often rushed and cut short because homework awaits. This is also a place and time where children have the opportunity to learn social and etiquette skills.

Sara Bennett and Nancy Kalish, coauthors of *The Case Against Homework*, interviewed dozens of families about the ill effects of homework on their lives. They found that for the sake of completing assignments, meal times together—an important time to reconnect and bond—are cut short. Families often give up leisure activities, social gatherings, recreation, after-school activities, trips and outings to places of interest, reading for fun, and time just being together as a family.[5]

To be sure, the stress that children feel about homework is contributing to negative attitudes about school. Alfie Kohn, a well-known educator and parenting expert, has combed through and analyzed much of the research out there on homework and has compiled his findings into numerous articles and a book devoted to this subject. There is overwhelming evidence challenging the myth that homework improves academic performance, raises test scores, or improves learning.

He quotes this statement released by the American Educational Research Association decades ago: "Whenever homework crowds out social experience, outdoor recreation, and creative activities, and whenever it usurps time that should be devoted to sleep, it is not meeting the basic needs of children and adolescents."

Additionally, he states that no study has ever confirmed the belief that homework generates nonacademic benefits, such as perseverance, independence, self-discipline, and time management skills—tools so critical for success. Furthermore, less positive attitudes toward school and learning are present in kids who get more assignments.[6]

While it is becoming more and more clear that excessive homework is potentially harmful, carefully planned assignments that have meaning and relevance to students in higher grades are seen by some as worthwhile. When homework content reinforces learning and helps retain interest in what students are learning, there seems to be less ground for negativity to take root. Busy work, on the other hand, can breed annoyance and resentment.[7]

A top-heavy workload is challenging enough for ten months out of the year. Nevertheless, in recent years, it has become the norm to give children summer assignments, too. Gone for many are the carefree days of summer when kids could feel free to explore their own interests, read books of their choosing, or just have time to themselves. Now they have assignments hanging over their heads, robbing them of the mental break from school they deserve and need after working so hard throughout the year.

How would we feel as adults if, after working a full day, we were required to put in overtime every evening, on weekends, and over vacations? Recreation, leisure activities, and time spent with friends and family are forfeited. Some of us know all too well how this feels. Careers, bosses, and supervisors may require it. Technology enables it. We may even impose this on ourselves. Regardless of the source, this is the definition of a *workaholic*.

When we frame it in this light, requiring kids to grow up living this kind of existence seems incredibly harsh, unfair, and irresponsible. Let's hope, in the very near future, we will acquire the sense to look back and say, "What were we *thinking*?" And then, for starters, offer our children our deepest apologies.

Remember back to chapter 1 when we discussed the purposes of blinking. It's useful to think about this from a physiological perspective, but it is also a metaphor. If kids work so hard to focus throughout the year, and vacation is their time to blink, how is this helping them to retain the ability to focus in September?

When a sampling of school administrators were asked for an explanation of the perceived benefits of summer homework, the reasons given included the following:

Summer assignments have been required for several years. There are many schools that require summer assignments for upper-level courses such as honors and advanced placement. Some of the benefits are:

- Helping students to remain focused on academics throughout the summer to prepare for the next school year. Often, important information is forgotten during the summer months. Working on summer assignments will help to retain the information.
- Summer assignments allow students to prepare for the expectations for honors and advanced placement courses so they are able to begin the school year with the correct focus regarding the rigor of the courses.
- Summer reading assignments for all levels allows students to continue reading during the summer months so that they do not become stagnant, and are ready for the expectations and requirements of the courses when they return in September.
- The College Board determines the pacing for Advanced Placement courses and it is often necessary for students enrolling in AP courses to begin lessons in the summer to ensure that teachers are able to cover all of the required materials prior to AP exams in May of each year.

Adding insult to injury is the increasingly normative practice of giving homework assignments over holiday breaks during the school year as well. Given what we now know about how homework overload is impacting children's mental and physical health, shouldn't we be questioning the set of expectations that dictate how much a child needs to know—in fact, how much information a child is capable of absorbing and retaining?

Challenge Success is a program affiliated with the Stanford Graduate School of Education that grew out of concern for the emotional and academic problems children were increasingly exhibiting in the United States. Child and adolescent experts spanning the fields of education, medicine, psychology, public health, and policy combined expertise and set out to devise new ways to help students achieve success and regain balance in their lives. They explore the homework issue in depth and strive to achieve a balanced viewpoint on its merits and drawbacks.

The goals of the program are twofold. The first involves reaching out to schools, parents, and communities to provide innovative support in dealing with what have become commonplace, everyday pressures that are stressing out students, whole families, and school environments. The second aim of the program is to research how these measures are having an influence on kids. Such new insights can help shape future policy decisions about how we educate our children.[8]

Sleep deprivation is another major concern. This is fortunately receiving new levels of attention even as of this writing. We know that adequate sleep is one of the most important factors contributing to our health and well-being, and this fact is, thankfully too, beginning to get its due. Yet time and again as parents we are forced to choose what our children should do: either sacrifice sleep so they can get all their work done, or risk having their grades affected by limiting how much our kids should do based on what our common sense is telling us.

When did it become customary to ignore a child's cries of fatigue because schools will not accept, *and respect*, a child's innate physical and mental limits?

In reality, their grades may be affected either way. Studies have shown that getting fewer than the recommended hours of sleep on a consistent basis lowers grades as well as cognitive functioning. What does increase are stress levels and anxiety. Squeezed out of daily life are the behaviors that would promote health and well-being and counter stress, but there isn't time because the homework demands are so great. It is a counterproductive, counterintuitive, vicious cycle that is causing harm and ultimately not helping our kids achieve better.[9]

Fortunately, parental instincts are getting some backup. As reported in a February 2015 issue of *Science Daily*, the National Sleep Foundation issued new recommendations for appropriate amounts of sleep in every age category. These findings are the result of collaboration among experts in the fields of sleep research, anatomy and physiology, pediatrics, neurology, gerontology, and gynecology, which had the goal of representing consensus from a wide range of specialty areas.

The bottom line is the recommended sleep ranges for most age groups were widened. They are now the following:

Newborns (0–3 months): Sleep range narrowed to 14–17 hours each day (previously it was 12–18)
Infants (4–11 months): Sleep range widened two hours to 12–15 hours (previously it was 14–15)

Toddlers (1–2 years): Sleep range widened by one hour to 11–14 hours (previously it was 12–14)

Preschoolers (3–5): Sleep range widened by one hour to 10–13 hours (previously it was 11–13)

School–age children (6–13): Sleep range widened by one hour to 9–11 hours (previously it was 10–11)

Teenagers (14–17): Sleep range widened by one hour to 8–10 hours (previously it was 8.5–9.5)

Younger adults (18–25): Sleep range is 7–9 hours (new age category)

Adults (26–64): Sleep range did not change and remains 7–9 hours

Older adults (65+): Sleep range is 7–8 hours (new age category)

Response to this landmark study can be summed up in the following quote: "This is the first time that any professional organization has developed age-specific recommended sleep durations based on a rigorous, systematic review of the world scientific literature relating sleep duration to health, performance and safety," says Charles A. Czeisler, PhD, MD, chairman of the board of the National Sleep Foundation, chief of sleep and circadian disorders at Brigham and Women's Hospital, and Baldino Professor of Sleep Medicine at the Harvard Medical School.

He adds, "The National Sleep Foundation is providing these scientifically grounded guidelines on the amount of sleep we need each night to improve the sleep health of the millions of individuals and parents who rely on us for this information."[10]

After decades of research exploring the effects that sleep has on our health, behavior, and functioning, a new groundbreaking study published in *Psychology Today* provides evidence that sleep does indeed affect learning and memory. Scientists from New York University and Peking University Shenzhen in China teamed up to design a study with the goal of actually observing changes in the brain that occur during sleep. The long-held hypothesis has been that "some strengthening of connections between neurons occurs, along with some pruning of synapses that help establish memories."

The study was successful in enabling them to actually observe changes in synapses after sleep, giving support to this hypothesis. Dr. Joseph A. Buckhalt explains:

> This new study builds importantly on a large body of literature that shows the importance of sleep for children. From birth, children spend much of their waking hours learning new information and skills. Infants sleep long hours and now it is clear that sleep is more than just "rest." Active reprocessing of neuronal connections takes place during sleep. As children get older, their learning continues, as does their need for sleep. We have known for some time that sufficient sleep is vital for optimal learning, and we continue to attain better understanding of the underlying mechanisms of *how* sleep facilitates learning. [11]

With regard to the sleep needs of teenagers, Google this subject and you will find no shortage of research that clearly indicates we are short-changing our teens' potential by overloading their physiological need for sleep with out-of-sync schedules and excessive workloads. Studies of circadian rhythms across age groups have shown that the sleep timetable shifts in adolescence. While this biological process has been known for some time, external factors influencing sleep patterns and outcomes are attracting more recent attention.

Whereas teens experience intrinsic developmental changes that affect their sleep behavior, our way of life is not structured to support this most basic human need. The demands of school, extracurricular activities, sports involvement, employment, and volunteer opportunities—all considered to be essential pursuits in the quest for college acceptance—vie for attention and strain the tired teen's stamina. When considering this dynamic and vulnerable juncture in the span of human development, it begs us to tune in and concern ourselves with the short-term and long-term effects.

Dr. Mary Carskadon, professor of psychiatry and human behavior at Brown University School of Medicine, puts this in cogent perspective. As reported in "When Worlds Collide—Adolescent Need for Sleep Versus Societal Demand," an article summarizing her research, she states, "Given that the primary focus of education is to maximize human potential, then a new task before us is to ensure that the conditions in which learning takes place address the very biology of our learners."

Delayed school start times are slowly making their way through school districts around the country. While this is a good start, she insightfully points out:

> Moving the opening bell to a later time may help many teens with the mismatch between biological time and scholastic time, but it will not provide more hours in the day. It is not difficult to project that a large number of students see a later starting time as permission to stay up later at night studying, working, surfing the net, watching television, and so forth. Today's teens know little about their sleep needs or about the biological timing system. Interestingly, students do know they are sleepy, but they do not have skills to cope with the issue, and many assume—just as adults do—that they are expected to function with an inadequate amount of sleep. This assumption is a physiological fallacy; sleep is not optional. Sleep is biologically obligatory.

In a progressive approach, she challenges us to create additional solutions. Just as we teach children about the importance of proper nutrition and healthy eating habits, so too, she encourages, should sleep education be included in the curriculum at every level. The subject of sleep requirements, patterns, and the science behind them affords infinite, exciting opportunities for cross-curricular development and implementation. [12]

So what would it take to get our education and health-care values in sync, so that learning can become a humane, nurturing experience as opposed to a stress-inducing, physically depleting one? This is a profoundly critical question, and one that deserves a prompt, constructive answer.

Many educators would argue that it is a much greater investment in the future lives of our children and the future life of our society to invest our time efficiently and design our curricula wisely, so that rather than focusing on trying to teach kids everything, we instead ignite their curiosity and passion for learning so they will grow into lifelong learners.

In effect, our children are barometers for our future. Their experiences reflect the pressure of modern life. If we pay attention, and look closely at the problems and challenges they are facing that are unique to this generation, we can clue into where the imbalances are and what we must do in order to fix them. Children are losing their childhoods, and this is nothing short of absolutely tragic. They are being overworked because school demands this of them, which is a response to the demands of our society. We are all caught up in a way of life that values getting ahead despite the detriment to our personal well-being.

As skill requirements have trickled down to lower and lower grade levels, the innate developmental stages that children progress though are being ignored. Social, emotional, and physical developmental needs are receiving less attention because there is a greater emphasis on academics. We know better. This will only cause bigger problems for children as they progress through school without building these skills, so necessary for success in all areas of life, at the appropriate time in the scope of their education.

We all have the same number of hours in the day that we did a generation ago. Yet the amount of information at our disposal, with options for communication and access to knowledge, is virtually limitless. This has influenced, some believe, our society's expectations of just how much information our children are being expected to learn—in the same number of hours and calendar days. Just look at their backpacks—the load they need to carry began requiring wheels a long time ago.

The irony of all this is our kids will be enormously depleted before they get the chance to lead the harried lives of their parents and bring up the next generation. Do we want to perpetuate the cycle? All to what end? And what do we do about it? How we find—or create—our niche in the global village and equip our children so they will be prepared to find their own niche in the world is no easy task.

We owe it to them, however, to imagine the possibilities if we do and to be committed to finding solutions to the problems that will keep us from getting there. And we must confront the potential consequences if we do not.

Let's reason that it begins with redefining our values, beginning with recognizing the priceless worth of our essential needs and prioritizing what really matters in our lives. Balance these answers with our existing time, energy, and resources and we just may come to our senses as a civilization. Then, its youngest and most vulnerable members may get the chance to grow up healthy and whole. The choice is collectively ours. We owe it to our children to choose wisely.

If we steer clear of the cultural clutter that zaps our inborn common sense, we might rediscover that we are, when all is said and done, *sensory beings*. Yet learning has become desensitized. In fact, daily living has become desensitized. Many of us have been conditioned, perhaps without being fully aware of it, that getting our needs met comes with a price. What exactly does it cost us? In essence, our own sense of wellness. Adults may have become immune to the degrading effects of this price tag, but it's heartbreaking to see how it's impacting our children.

Wellness is, as defined in the *Oxford English Dictionary*, "the state or condition of being in good physical, mental, and spiritual health, especially as an actively pursued goal."[13] Wellness is likely first on our list of life's priorities. Without this, nothing else of value really manifests or matters. So what does it take to achieve wellness?

We know the simple answers: adequate rest, exercise, healthy food choices, healthy relationships, and the ability to find balance in our lives. We feel balanced when we are able to meet our goals, feel a sense of fulfillment, and have fun along the way. Yet reaching equilibrium can be far from simple. Much of it comes down to the idea of sustainability, and it does so on many levels that are intricately connected.

The problems our children, families, schools, and communities are facing have become so prevalent that it is becoming less and less feasible for schools to meet our children's needs and for families to provide the extra support their kids require.

"Specifically, child study teams (CSTs) have made a well-meaning effort to address an ever-widening number of factors that are impacting our kids mentally, physically, and emotionally," states Dr. Linda Tamm, a psychologist in private practice. "Unfortunately, CSTs are overwhelmed due to steadily increasing numbers of children who need to be evaluated. Screenings have become broader in scope because the time it takes to complete the process, and the staff needed to implement it, are overburdened."

She sums it up with a metaphor that evokes a great visual. "CST evaluations have become bigger nets, and a lot is falling through the bigger holes that come with bigger nets."

The causes of this are complex. For example, there has been an explosion of AD/HD and autism diagnoses. Additionally, the legal classification of academic disabilities has opened up to include many different types of diagnoses, including special physical circumstances such as Lyme disease and chronic fatigue syndrome.

The *DSM-IV*, long considered to be the "bible" for mental health-care practitioners, has gone through some changes in the past year. Aside from its new name, the *DSM-V*, it changed its criteria for a learning disability diagnosis. It also removed the term *Asperger's* from its list of diagnoses. It has been replaced by supplementary diagnoses that characterize specific parts of the disorder instead of one cohesive descriptor.

"The new criteria for learning disorders is much broader, requiring simply exhibiting problems in performance for six months and not re-sponding to typical interventions," explains Dr. Tamm. "One has to prove 'difficulties' with performance or understanding that can then be confirmed by testing that is standardized. While we celebrate a growing understanding of the ways kids can fall behind and deserve help, this tool still doesn't address the causes, like visual impairments."

This approach also focuses on documenting the *consequences* of im-pairments, she further explains, but it does not define the *causes*. "Of-ten how a child behaves during testing as compared to in the classroom, or subtle differences that come out between two sub-tests, can reveal a visual deficit. However, that requires great attention to detail, as well as time, to compare the results between the psychologist, learning consul-tant, and teacher. The answer is in the data and the staff experience, but it is lost without the right questions being asked."

And of course, the staff must be equipped with knowledge about visual deficits in the first place. If these types of learning problems are not on their radar, the right questions will certainly not be asked. With the numbers of kids who are affected by these being what they are, and the holes in the net being the size that they are, you now understand the reason for the subtitle of this book. We are losing an enormous number of kids through these holes.

CSTs are trying hard to be more accommodative by providing an-swers and support for the many conditions with which kids are strug-gling. Still, with the scales tipped as they are—with need outweighing support—the finer points of evaluation results may not get attention simply because there just isn't time to look closely enough at the find-ings. It's time to weave a new net.

The takeaway here for parents and teachers is this: just because a CST evaluation doesn't turn up answers or a diagnosis doesn't mean there aren't any. Seek out another opinion, or two, and keep looking. Include a behavioral optometrist in your search. This may be the stone left unturned that unleashes the answer, or at least one of them. There are many, though, who don't know that this stone exists. Now that you do, pass it on.

It's important to reiterate that if the child did receive a diagnosis, having them evaluated by a behavioral optometrist should be part of the process going forward. Looking for visual causes and doing vision therapy if it is recommended will make a difference. Leaving this piece out, if a visual deficit is present, will leave the child still struggling no matter what other intervention is brought in.

It's of interest to mention that the establishment of compulsory education in the early 1900s coincides with the detection of vision-related learning problems. [14] That's not to say that these disorders first came about with the existence of this new educational model. It may very well be that visual deficits have invariably been present over the course of human history, pre-dating any research. On this we can only speculate.

Factor in that in earlier times our lifestyles were shaped by daily activities that centered on meeting our basic needs for food, clothing, and shelter. We didn't focus at near-point distances for concentrated periods of time like we do now. However, the structured, routinized archetype of education that has been central from the early 1900s up to the present day may have provided an agent through which these disorders became recognizable.

It may also be inducing them. Dr. Barry Tannen, a behavioral optometrist and associate clinical professor at SUNY College of Optometry, lectures widely about vision-related learning problems and vision therapy. He shared an unsettling observation, noting that he is seeing more and more fifth and sixth graders walk through his door with symptoms and, ultimately, in need of vision therapy. What he finds particularly unsettling, though, is the increased number of children in earlier grades (1–3) who are presenting with visual symptoms more typical of older students.

Why this increase? In her book *Eyes for Learning*, Dr. Antonia Orfield cites many reasons for this from her perspective and firsthand experience as a behavioral optometrist. A former classroom teacher, Dr.

Orfield was inspired to pursue a career in this field after vision therapy helped her overcome extreme nearsightedness that had progressed from childhood and left her feeling unsafe even to drive later on in adulthood.

Dr. Orfield's experience as a teacher and mother, who took her own children to Dr. Amiel Francke for vision therapy, enabled her to make a distinctive connection between vision and learning. This unparalleled view guided her in her treatment of children and motivated her to reach out beyond the walls of her practice to help others understand the importance of supporting healthy vision development.

Dr. Orfield understood, from a rational holistic point of view, how vision is impacted by everything around us and in us. This includes sleep and movement patterns, nutrition, exposure to stressors and toxins of all kinds, and the home and school environments.

One stressor that our children encounter very early on that we are likely not attuned to and "desperately needs more research," according to Dr. Orfield, is the size of print children are expected to read in the early grades. "Too many bright children are failing reading, and others are going myopic (nearsighted) from adaptations to small print at close distances too early in their visual development," she writes. In addition to print size, the distance of reading material from their eyes is also in need of attention. Being forced to focus up close before the visual system is mature enough can interfere with visual development and cause problems. [15]

Compounding these existing developmentally inappropriate stressors is the looming presence and allure of screens. Dr. Orfield incisively recognizes, "What many behavioral optometrists know from experience with patients is that computer time needs to be limited until children truly need it by age nine for school, and even then, very infrequent use is the ideal until eighth or ninth grade. Fourth graders I see for therapy are being required to turn in homework done on the computer. Our culture has not learned to use its inventions wisely, and knowledge of the side effects of electronic media is not widespread." [16]

These were her words in 2007. Nine years later, we are witness to an unprecedented increase in our usage of screens for learning, testing, and communication. Tablets and laptops are regular fixtures in classrooms at younger and younger ages. How is this affecting children's development? I would add to Dr. Orfield's comment about the limited knowledge of side effects the notion that we won't fully understand technology's impact on development and learning outcomes for decades. This is another area in need of intensive study.

The relationship of the body with the surrounding environment, and even within itself, has great bearing on learning outcomes. Dr. Darell Harmon's pioneering research contributed landmark insights into the interaction of posture, body mechanics, gravity, lighting, classroom furniture design, and the distance between reading material and the eyes. His collaborative nine-year study involving 160,000 children showed remarkable findings about conditions under which children learn.[17]

Lighting conditions, including intensity reflecting off work surfaces as well as glare, can cause children to instinctively adjust their body positioning to relieve the stress that this creates on the eyes. In doing so, this affects more than just their posture. Harmon called these adjustments "body mechanics," which accounted for not only the alignment of the spine while sitting but also "the torque, force and compression of the intervertebral discs of the spine."

From here there is a domino-like effect that impacts the body on both large and small scales. Muscles and bones are thrown off balance. Since the spine is the main highway for communication throughout the entire nervous system, the chemistry of the body as well as the neural functioning is altered due to the warping of the spine.

And not surprisingly, the eyes and capacity for visual processing are compromised. To remedy this, he designed desktops that can be raised to a 20 percent angle. This reduced the need to position the body awkwardly to relieve the glare on the eyes, eased the strain on the spine, and allowed for gaze to fall at a proper angle and eliminate the stress on the visual system. Dr. Harmon was so in tune with the interrelationship between posture and vision, he was known to be able to observe someone's back from behind as the person walked and know what prescription that person would need for his or her glasses.

Desk height is another factor that ultimately affects visual dexterity. As is common, the accommodation that the body must make to fit into this personal physical workspace that is framed by the boundaries of the furniture can cause strain, leading to fatigue. When the larger muscles tire out, it becomes more challenging to resist gravity and remain in a balanced postural position.

Flat work surfaces put stress on the neck muscles, as they must hold up the head in a bent-over position. Awkward head positioning changes the angles at which the eyes focus on close-up material. In turn, this can distort the information coming in through the eyes to the brain. Ultimately, this can interfere with proper visual development. Dr. Harmon was able to document correlations between specific visual dysfunctions and environmental conditions.

The slanted desktop was a partial answer to this, allowing for the head and neck to be positioned at an angle that puts the least amount of strain on the supporting muscles in response to gravitational pull, in addition to reducing the glare factor. Besides this, the "Harmon distance," as it became known, is characterized as the distance from the first knuckle to the elbow and is used as a measurement when referring to optimal learning conditions. This would be the ideal distance between the eyes and the visual task.[18]

Screens aside, the elements of learning environments addressed in Harmon's research alone are enough to cause distress to a developing body's mutually dependent functions. Concluding that "the body is involved in the entire process of vision," he advocated for providing proper chair and desk heights, prioritizing good lighting, and monitoring healthy posture. Dr. Harmon's research conclusions and recommendations are rich fodder for education reform.

Addressing the surplus of modern stressors that plague everyone who is tethered to a desk because their work requires it, whether it is a first grader or an office worker, Drs. Amiel Francke and Walter Kaplan point out the importance of a comfortable workspace. "This article is a uniquely optometric public service," begins the abstract summarizing the article they coauthored titled "Easier and More Productive Study and Desk Work."

Timing, location, lighting, and physical positioning are usually out of our control given that we are typically bound by a set schedule and space. However, these are very important aspects of our experience as workers and can even affect the quality of our experiences and the work we produce. How we feel in response to our surroundings is also considered important. Room temperature, the presence of fresh air circulating, noise, clutter, and even our clothing are factors that influence us and deserve attention. Breaks, exercise, and stretching are essential.

While they recognize that it may be difficult or impossible to arrange for all the pieces to be in place to create an optimal learning environment, striving to include as many as possible can help maximize productivity.[19]

All of these external factors are important. The internal details are, too. These are overlooked, however, when it comes to defining—and mandating—what children are expected to learn and when. Despite the fact that children's sensory systems are not fully equipped and ready to handle the requirements made of them in the early years of school, we override this because some think this will *make* kids learn. In truth, this stance is interfering with developmental processes that are unfolding naturally, which are what will actually ready them for learning. We can't force this. Yet in blindly doing so, we are not only disturbing their development, but we may also be inducing problems that will inhibit their ability to learn as they mature.

Dr. Hannaford explains why it is crucial to understand these internal details and why children are not *biologically* ready to read before the age of seven.

"Light passes across the body of the eyeball onto the retina where 137 million nerve receptors (nerve endings) take in the information. Ninety-five percent of the receptors, the rods, are for peripheral vision, while only five percent are cones for foveal focus, which is what we use for up close, two-dimensional paper work."

Why is this significant?

"Before entering school, three-dimensional and peripheral vision allow the greatest environmental learning. They integrate the visual with the kinesthetic to understand shapes, movement of natural forms and spatial awareness. When children enter school, they are often expected to quickly develop their foveal focus in order to see small, static, two-dimensional letters on a page. The transition from three-dimensional and peripheral to foveal focus is very abrupt and in many cases unnatural," she elucidates.

Before approximately age seven, the ciliary bodies (muscles that shape the lens of the eye) are short, causing the lens to be thin and elongate. With the lens in this shape, the incoming image is spread out across the retina, bringing into play maximum rod and cone stimulation. The lens shape easily accommodates three-dimensional, peripheral and distance vision. At about age seven, these muscles start to lengthen, allowing the lens to round out and more easily focus the image only on the fovea centralis of the retina for natural foveal focus. Children who have looked at books in the home may have already acquired some foveal focus if the process was their choice and free of stress and pressure to perform, however, most children are not physically ready to read at age five as is now mandated in our schools.[20]

In addition to this, she explains that by age seven or eight, motor coordination and brain maturation synchronize along with eye muscle control, allowing for eye teaming and binocular vision to come about naturally.[21] It is a stunning, awe-inspiring progression. The human brain prepares to learn about the world even while in utero. The vestibular system goes into action from the moment of conception. Responding to gravity and movement, this system coordinates with the brain, core muscles, and the eyes, creating a foundational mechanism for learning.[22]

We tend to think of vision and visual functioning as a local task. "Vision is a very complex phenomenon, with only a small percentage (less than five percent) of the process occurring in the eyes. The other ninety-five percent of vision takes place in the brain from association with touch, hearing and proprioception," explains Dr. Hannaford.

Even when we acknowledge the involvement of the brain, we are still concentrating our attention to learning within the vicinity of the head. Yet we know now that vision is dependent and influential upon the entire body. A growing body of research is showing that movement improves academic achievement and brain function and helps hone visual ability.[23]

Stress of any kind that can affect us in various ways can also impinge on vision. Lifestyle practices, including nutrition, sleep hygiene, sedentary versus active routines, and the wide-ranging demands of school, can overwhelm kids and cause imbalances to play out in any of the physical, emotional, and psychosocial realms. Another surprising effect on vision involves the stress response. When one senses danger, the reflexive response that moves the eyes outward to see what threat is looming greatly impedes the ability of the eyes to team and track along a line of print. If a child lives in chronic stressful conditions, this can affect the child's eye muscles and make it hard to focus and track.[24]

While we all experience stress at times, which can even be helpful in motivating our actions, undue amounts of stress can diminish quality of life. This is tragic when it affects innocent children who are bursting with energy, curiosity, excitement, and wonder.

Presently, we are witness to a stirring period in educational history as ongoing questions, debate, criticism, and attempts to transform schools and learning environments continue to draw attention, deservedly so. There is much that needs fixing.

Beyond the need for repair, there is also much that needs healing. Fixing and healing are two different things. Fixing what's broken is an immediate action in response to a need stemming from a flaw that causes dysfunction. Healing is the process of restoring wellness, balance, and wholeness to that which suffered injury or disorder inflicted by the brokenness.

Education needs healing. Above and beyond this, however, is the poignant truth that our children need healing even more. Knowledge and awareness are powerful tools, but only when they are put to good use. Recognizing that there are answers to learning problems that have escaped explanation for so long is without a doubt a welcome revelation. Taking action to remedy these problems can be life changing. Blazing new trails toward an approach to educating our kids in ways that will support them in their full development rather than work against them may not only benefit individual lives, but perhaps even initiate a cultural renaissance.

6

CHANGING LIVES

Making a World of Difference

Remember Janie's story from chapter 3, the second grader who revealed to her teachers that the letters on the paper "moved all by themselves"? After celebrating the huge clue they had just been given, the sting of reality set in as Janie's teachers felt themselves hit a wall together because they both knew they were powerless to do anything with this information.

They speculated they'd find much-needed answers to Janie's struggles if a comprehensive vision exam were included in the evaluation plan developed by the child study team. Currently, however, this is not standard practice.

Here is a gray area so huge we could lose the elephant in the room in it. Along with the elephant, we are also losing our kids.

Comprehensive vision exams and vision therapy should be seen as just as worthy of funding as other support therapies provided for by school districts. We need to establish a universal understanding that vision requires attention in the sphere of education with regard to children's developmental needs.

The huge struggles that children go through have far-reaching effects on their lives. It is easy to see how they can be easily misdiagnosed, wrongly placed in a system that is unequipped to deal with the real problem, even medicated, with the tragic outcome of never actually being rehabilitated despite all these measures. The intentions are good, but we're missing the mark for pure lack of information.

Vision is so integral to learning yet does not receive uniform acknowledgment, attention, and support in the majority of learning environments. It is time for this to change. Our practices must catch up with our vast stores of acquired knowledge about child development. Surely we can connect the dots for ourselves and understand how a life trajectory can unfold for a struggling child.

Dr. William Moskowitz once said that knowledge about vision-related learning problems will change lives and change the world. Indeed, he maintained, it may even save lives. There is great depth to his words.

Most certainly a child who is struggling academically will face challenges emotionally, socially, and psychologically. Self-esteem erodes in the face of such constant strain. Frustration sets in when a student is trying yet still failing, which can eventually lead to rebellious and deviant behavior. Tragically, individual lives can fall through the cracks when the real problem at the root of a child's struggles goes unrecognized.

According to research carried out through the former Catalyst Vision and Learning Program, the inability to read is the largest common denominator among juvenile delinquents.[1] Vision problems affect 66 percent of illiterate adults, 70 percent of juvenile delinquents, and 75 percent of prisoners. These strained lives affect society. This is why educating the community about the connection between visual deficits and criminal behavior is key, in the words of the late Margie Thompson, founder of P.A.V.E., Parents Active for Vision Education. Margie was a visionary, and her advocacy work was pioneering.

Children who are struggling in school will be faced with a cascade of secondary difficulties as a result of the sheer exertion they put forth in their attempts to keep up with demands. Behavior and attention problems can be present in the early grades and even beforehand, during the preschool years. Parents may attribute these challenges to any number of causes. Some will be identified, and some won't. Some will figure out only part of the whole picture.

From here children enter school at a disadvantage. They may already be acquiring a negative self-image, which, in addition to their struggles, will complicate matters for them. Self-fulfilling prophecy sets a downward spiral in motion, and the stage is set for failure. Behavior problems may trump learning problems, and classification and/or medication is coming down the pike. Sadly, children's self-esteem is eroding, and they are filled with negative feelings about school and, worst of all, about themselves. [2]

Giving up on oneself is tragic, yet this bleak reality is what so many children live with day in and day out. Unquestionably, getting through each day must feel like a survival situation. They look around and wonder why it seems so easy for others. They feel defective and doubt themselves and their future. In an attempt to gain acceptance and belonging during these critical formative years of their life, they seek recognition in other ways.

Embarrassment and shame are powerful motivators in the very worst sense. For children who aren't succeeding in school, repeatedly falling short of the goal line can feel out of their control, which is very uncomfortable. To relieve this tension, they will focus on succeeding with something that is in their control, such as distracting attention away from the daily activities that expose their failures. When success is eluding kids through conventional measures, deviant tactics may take up residence.

Aberrant behavior can be a red flag.

Disruptive behavior, rebelliousness, defiance, rejecting authority, withdrawal, and isolation are examples of behavioral outcomes of this sad scenario. These actions may lead to emotional, social, and psychological problems. Clamoring to cope, kids may turn to drug and alcohol use, truancy, skipping school altogether, and eventually to criminal behavior. The root of the problem has been sorely missed, and they have begun a descent into a lifelong battle with themselves and the laws and expectations of society.

Thoughts and feelings are the driving forces behind behavior. Behavior can be a symptom of a bigger problem that may go unchecked. Unfortunately, all too often what lies beneath is left undiscovered in children who are attracting so much negative attention because of their deviant actions. The adults in their life, whether these are a parent, teacher, counselor, or coach, grasp at whatever resources are available and within reach to try to handle the behavior and its effects. Limitations of time, money, energy, and answers to the problem are realities that can encumber this effort.

Vision-related learning problems are present in the general population in epidemic proportions. In the juvenile delinquent (JD) population alone, they are present in the majority of young offenders.[3]

One of the earliest studies in this realm dates back to 1949. Optometrist Dr. David Dzik found that 91 percent of the population in a Tennessee juvenile facility tested below grade level. Further visual testing revealed that nearly all of those participants in the study had a vision-related learning problem.[4] Dr. Dzik's work was considered groundbreaking. In an article published in the January 5, 1968, issue of *The Optometric Weekly*, he points to the rising crime rate and the tens of billions of dollars this costs the United States. The increase of delinquency, he acknowledged, makes "it more and more clear that something must be done."

In this article he shares the following statement from the President's Commission on Law Enforcement and Administration of Justice, established by President Johnson on July 23, 1965: "The high degree of correlation between delinquency and failure in school is more than accidental."[5]

We've come a long way in our understanding of this connection since then. Equipped with the knowledge we now have about learning, along with the increasing multitude of diagnoses for learning challenges, juxtaposed to the escalation of violent crimes committed by children, especially when they're carried out in a school setting, the question beckons—how much real progress have we made? Have we answered the plea made by Dr. Dzik that something must be done?

Some alarming statistics compiled four decades ago that emerged from Dr. Dzik's work include the following findings from research done with children at the Hamilton County Juvenile Court in Chattanooga, Tennessee:

- Of the 125 children tested in early 1965, 94 percent failed the reading and comprehension tests.
- Of 111 children tested between January and May 1967 for reading and comprehension, 90 percent were from one to seven grade levels below actual grade level.
- Seventy-four percent of children administered vision screening tests failed one or more tests in 1965.

- Over 70 percent of children screened failed one or more of the vision tests between 1966 and 1967.
- Over $40,000,000 per year is the cost incurred to educate first through sixth graders who repeat a grade in school in Tennessee.[6]

Additional studies spanning several decades beyond Dr. Dzik's initial look at JD populations, by behavioral optometrists and lead researchers Dr. Paul Harris and Dr. Stan Kaseno, showed the percentage of offenders with vision-related learning problems averaged 94 percent.[7]

Undetected vision problems were found in 74 percent of adjudicated adolescents as of 2000, and a 2003 national assessment of prison inmates found that only 43 percent had graduated from high school or earned an equivalency diploma prior to being incarcerated.[8]

In his 1974 address to the World Congress on Dyslexia cosponsored by the Orton Society and the Mayo Clinic, Peter D. Wright presented his reviews of the literature linking learning disabilities and juvenile delinquency. The North Carolina Crime Study Commission conducted its own study, intrigued after Wright shared related research conducted by Dr. Dennis Hogenson with the assistant attorney general in Virginia.[9]

The first two paragraphs of their report, *Learning Disabilities and Their Relation to Crime and Delinquency*, read as follows:

> In attempting to formulate comprehensive crime prevention programs over the years, innumerable study commissions, blue ribbon panels, penologists, investigative agencies, and other experts in all phases of the criminal justice field have grappled with the problem of identifying the primary underlining causes of crime and delinquency. The Crime Study Commission is cognizant of and concurs with many of the most recent efforts which have found such factors as (1) deprived socio-economic status, (2) unemployment, (3) poor school performance, (4) broken homes and (5) mental illness, as being primary contributing factors.
>
> The Crime Study Commission in this report will attempt to go one step further in the search for the cause of crime by postulating a theory, which simply stated, will argue that, "reading failure is the single most significant factor in those forms of delinquency which can be described as anti-socially aggressive." If we believe that a significant amount of serious crime is committed by individuals who

began their anti-social behavior as school dropouts and who graduated from juvenile delinquents to youthful offenders to adult criminals,
then this theory, if proven, becomes a vitally important indicator for
crime prevention.

Wright restated the compelling statement made by the commission
and it bears repeating here too: "Reading failure is the single most
significant factor in those forms of delinquency which can be described
as anti-socially aggressive." Yet despite this insight, we still haven't
made tangible strides with remediation.

Wright is also in a position to know the implications here. His extensive experience working with training schools and as a probation officer
in the court system has given him a close-up view of the many frustra-
tions he witnessed among the kids under his jurisdiction. Citing extensive research corroborating low reading levels with delinquency, Wright
makes the case for a child's right to an education with *the full support of
services* working in their favor, as opposed to against them.

In other words, society must recognize when kids are truly struggling
with an undiagnosed learning problem that is contributing to their
course of failure, first in the classroom and then out in the world. It is
our responsibility to acknowledge this and work toward implementing
solutions that will help remediate kids versus exacerbating their challenges. Education and justice systems must cooperate with the common
goal of supporting lasting measurable transformation in children whose
needs have gone unrecognized and unmet. They've already failed in the
educational system. They will remain trapped on a failing track in the
justice system unless they get the help they need. [10]

Twenty-five years ago, behavioral optometrists Treasure Wheeler
and Charles McQuarrie presented a paper at the National Academy of
Practices titled "Vision, Juvenile Delinquency and Learning Disabilities." They gave a comprehensive overview of the problem and what
was known then: "The link between learning disabilities and juvenile
delinquency has been established, as well as the link between vision and
learning disabilities." Based on compelling research findings, they stated clearly that school performance is a predominant forecaster of juvenile delinquency.

If A=B and B=C, then . . .

It was noted that while some offenders are testing social boundaries
or rebelling against authority, and move past this behavior as they ma-

ture, those who are struggling with a learning disability do not. They continue to decline. "The major concern is that uncompensated learning disabilities in delinquent youth lead to a recurrent cycle of destructive acts, whereas delinquents without learning disabilities tend to outgrow their delinquent ways," affirm Drs. Wheeler and McQuarrie.[11]

Research and exploration of the link between delinquency and learning disabilities continues to draw attention across disciplines. Dr. Paul Harris's research study titled "The Prevalence of Visual Conditions in a Population of Juvenile Delinquents" detected vision problems in just over 98 percent of the population tested at the Charles H. Hickey Jr. School in Baltimore County, Maryland. Dr. Harris emphasizes that optometry can and should play a major role in both diagnosing and treating such problems.[12]

Despite an array of rehabilitation services for juvenile offenders and prisoners while they are in confinement, success cases are limited. Lawyers who work in the juvenile system share a common view regarding what would improve kids' chances of not returning to the system—early intervention. In addition to rehabilitating deficient skill areas, such a proactive approach can also offer much hope. If we can construct the juvenile justice system to attend to these problems, minor offenders can get a second chance at building their lives.[13]

Building more prisons to contain those who are considered threats to society is not the answer. It is simply bandaging a fracture. As the fracture expands, it requires a bigger and bigger bandage. A better solution would be to provide support and restorative measures to what is broken, so it can heal. To do this, the correct diagnosis is needed in order to know what support and measures are required.[14]

It has been insightfully pointed out by optometrists themselves that visual rehabilitation is not a panacea for the range of problems with which juvenile offenders are struggling. By contrast, not every child who has a vision problem goes on to become a juvenile delinquent. ODs assert that a multidisciplinary approach to juvenile delinquents' rehabilitation is necessary.[15]

Citing the likely presence of a complicated combination of issues that can be involved with juvenile delinquency, Dr. Joel Zaba underscores the need for comprehensive care delivered in a team approach. "As we consider the issue of emotional problems leading to social problems and delinquency, we must again recognize that no single profession holds the key solution. When it comes to delinquency, we need appropriate counseling, court services, psychological services, educational and medical services, as well as basic optometric services."[16]

The important point is that all the ingredients are included in the mix. Given the importance of each, if any are left out, the treatment will be lacking and the outcome could be compromised. The vision piece, so vital yet often overlooked—albeit not even known—must become an established part of the whole rehabilitation process.

Enter a vision for the future—preventing vision-related learning problems early on by providing universal comprehensive vision examinations, so that all children who need help get help. Not only will this reduce the number of children who wind up in special education classes unnecessarily, or mistakenly medicated, it can prevent young lives from deteriorating and winding up incarcerated. In addition to the creation of a standard for vision evaluation programs in schools, additional preventive programs must be established for at-risk kids. This will require collaborative community organization. *The investment of time and resources is well worth it.*

Large-scale involvement is essential and must include families, schools, and the extended community.

While it may seem daunting, we do not have to reinvent the wheel. This idea has been well thought out over time by practitioners and experts who see the potential for saving lives and improving society. Included below are guidelines, developed by Drs. Wheeler and McQuarrie, which can be a model for implementation to work toward this goal.

Guidelines for Developing Juvenile Delinquency Preventive Programs

1. All state legislatures need to enact state laws requiring all juvenile delinquents to have a developmental vision evaluation upon intake.
2. Court Intake Forms should have a referral for vision evaluations.
3. Every state juvenile service should have an optometric consultant.
4. Each state training school should have an optometric consultant.
5. As an individual enters school and is repeatedly frustrated by the inability to learn by regular class approaches and methods, it

seems quite likely that some form of behavior problem might result. Schools should examine children at an early age to find the high risks for learning disability and refer for a behavioral vision evaluation.

6. States must require vision screening programs in primary grades that go beyond the Snellen 20/20.

7. Change Public Law 94-142 so that the schools can accomplish the job of eliminating visually-based learning disabilities that lead to juvenile problems. This will be accomplished by early identification of children who are visually at risk for failure in the classroom and the development of individual visual programs for children through the Individualized Education Plan (IEP) process.

8. Develop programs to promote community awareness and support through public education.

9. Provide preventive family counseling focusing on educating all members of the family to understand the learning-disabled juvenile delinquent. Many of the problems of the parents or siblings can be identified and handled, behavior management techniques can be implemented, dysfunctional family roles can be shifted, strategies for finding and getting the necessary help can be provided. The knowledge of what the learning-disabled delinquent goes through can be used to plan positive, rather than frustrating experiences at home and with peers.

Community Involvement: Developing a Referral Program

The preventive aspect of finding "at risk" children is to familiarize the child care service providers and community residents with the dynamics of the problem. It is necessary to disseminate information in seminars and workshops. These workshops should cover all aspects of learning-disabled juvenile delinquents, from how to identify the signs or behaviors of high-risk children to where and how to refer these children and their families.

Examples of community groups to be included:

1. Public health clinics
2. Public agencies
3. Preschool programs
4. Day care providers
5. Community health care providers
6. Community business and professional organizations

7. Fire departments
8. Law enforcement departments[17]

Studies have shown that vision therapy can play a pivotal role in the rehabilitation of an offender. Whereas there is often a host of issues needing attention in this process, the vision piece is so significant that leaving it out of the approach can limit the effectiveness of other treatment practices. Repeatedly, vision therapy was found to help these individuals overcome visual deficits, learn to read, and make conscious choices to turn their lives around and even pursue their education.

Dr. Joel Zaba has studied the presence of vision-related learning problems in this population for decades. His research findings have demonstrated that young criminal offenders who received vision therapy were six times less likely to have repeat offenses and return to the JD system than those offenders who did not receive treatment for their vision deficits.[18]

Think about this—as a society we can actually fight crime by rehabilitating vision and teaching prison and JD populations how to read. This constructive act of triage would address the current downfall of individual lives that may have fallen through the cracks for lack of information. It will give hope for new beginnings and a new start with newfound skills and capabilities.

As of a count in 2008, there were a total of 2,319,258 juvenile and adult inmates in U.S. local, state, and federal jails. This accounts for 1 in every 99.1 adults, and the numbers are on the rise along with the costs. With this increase, we can't afford not to make changes.[19]

In a highly regarded study that ran over an eleven-year time period, residents at the Regional Youth Education Facility in San Bernardino, California, participated in a rehabilitative vision program that included thorough vision evaluations and treatment. Seventy percent of those tested had displayed vision problems that interfered with learning. This action reduced the recidivism rate from over 45 percent to 16 percent or less every year over the course of the study, as reported in the 1989 California Department of Youth Authority report.[20]

Now think about this—we can actually reduce the crime rate going forward by restructuring our education system to not only treat vision problems in children but also prevent them in the first place. Some very forward-thinking studies have discussed the cost-effectiveness of funding this type of intervention for children as young as kindergarten age versus what it costs to give special education services to a child all throughout the child's schooling.

A 2008 study out of Teachers College, Columbia University, titled *Narrowing the Achievement Gap for Low-Income Children: A 19-Year Life Cycle Approach,* is a visionary example of how a holistic balance of measures can give disadvantaged children the care and support that can potentially enable them to grow up healthy and equipped to become successful learners and world citizens.

Taking into account the socioeconomic factors that impact a child's development, the limitations that ensue, and the stress that families feel as a result, this model proposes intervention spanning the prenatal stage all the way through the completion of high school. Support for mothers and families include prenatal and obstetrical care, family support, early childhood education, and pediatric care.

In addition, this model also includes support that extends outside the home. Adequate compensation for teachers who serve disadvantaged children and high-quality after-school and summer programs would help ensure that children receive academic, social, and creative stimulation in settings composed of low teacher-student ratios.

The designers of this proposed model, Drs. Tamara Wilder, Richard Rothstein, and Whitney Allgood, included comprehensive vision care alongside all other aspects of medical care. Comprehensive vision evaluation and vision therapy are included in the mix and seen as necessary ingredients. Indeed, if we are to address the whole child, we know this is vital. A progressive and all-encompassing model such as this holds promise for countless children who are in danger of falling through the cracks for any number of reasons.

The study sheds light on the human and economic advantages of investing dollars in services that would prevent problems and deficits from occurring, versus treating them after they have already taken a toll on a child's life, which, in turn, will take its toll on society. This realization is backed by the views and conclusions of top researchers cited in this study.

Dr. James Heckman, who won the 2000 Nobel Prize in Economics, along with colleagues Dr. Jack P. Shonkoff and Deborah Phillips, and who published *From Neurons to Neighborhoods,* a National Academy of Sciences study on early childhood neurobiological development, points out one of the primary inadequacies of public policy as it fails to recognize the long-term effects of academic failure and deficient socialization.

Underscoring that the achievement gap presents itself before a child enters school, they make clear the notion that school interventions are reactive—that is, they address already existing problems that require the child to catch up and go through compensatory measures to be on par. They highlight the superior alternative—taking proactive measures to prevent the gap from materializing into mammoth proportions in the first place.

More recently, Drs. Heckman and Shonkoff and their colleagues framed it as follows in the quoted head note they cited: "Skills beget skills, success breeds success, and the provision of positive experiences early in life is considerably less expensive and more effective than the cost and effectiveness of corrective intervention at a later age."[21]

The Head Start program is the outgrowth of initiatives launched in response to President Johnson's 1964 declaration of "The War on Poverty." Founded by Dr. Ed Zigler, a former faculty member of the Child Study Center at Yale University, it is a comprehensive program designed to provide preschool children with services that support their growth and development. Health and nutrition, parent engagement, education, social services, and special needs are the five components that make up the program.

"Head Start celebrated fifty years earlier this year and is one of the oldest federal programs to stay alive," states Dr. Marcy Guddemi. "Head Start is the best model out there."

Dr. Guddemi has summarized the effectiveness of the program and outlined its overall impact. The research data assessing the outcomes of Head Start intervention reveal, in some measure, a dependency upon the autonomous differences of individual programs, as well as the research focus. In other words, Head Start programs may vary in quality, therefore affecting outcomes. In addition, analysis of test scores can reflect a somewhat skewed picture. There is improvement in math and literacy in the early years up through third grade, but then improvements level off. This has led some to question its effectiveness.

However, looking beyond test scores is essential to recognizing and understanding the noteworthy successes of Head Start: less grade retention, less remediation, less juvenile delinquency, higher graduation rates, higher adult employment, and less incarceration. These "benefits to society," characterized by Dr. Guddemi, are priceless in that they represent the positive impact Head Start has on vulnerable young lives. When children are supported across the board, with their needs being thoroughly met, they are in a much better position to succeed.

When Charles Brittingham, former president of the Wilmington, Delaware, branch of the NAACP, learned about the far-reaching impact of vision-related learning problems on academic performance and achievement, and the success that vision therapy can have on their remediation, he took action. Amazed by the role these problems played in high school dropout rates, as well as prison and juvenile delinquent recidivism rates, he wrote a resolution that passed unanimously by the NAACP Delaware branch.

In addition to acknowledging that vision therapy can help reduce the high rate of recidivism, it urges members to "take aggressive action to have Vision Therapy included in all re-entry programs for formerly incarcerated persons." Determined and wanting more widespread awareness and knowledge of this, he brought the resolution to the national level. In 2009, the NAACP passed the *Resolution on Vision, Learning, and High-Risk Populations* at its 100th Anniversary National Convention in New York City.

The NAACP national resolution "calls for its members and units to educate the community, elected officials and correctional facilities about the merits of optometric vision therapy in helping to reduce the recidivism rate in some prisoners thereby increasing opportunities for persons reentering society."[22]

Taking proactive measures is ideal.

Thanks in part to the advocacy efforts of the American Optometric Association, the Affordable Care Act now includes this benefit for all children through eighteen years of age. Pediatric eye health care is deemed an "essential health benefit" and includes an annual comprehensive eye exam and treatment, which includes medical eye care and eyeglasses. Under this plan optometrists must be recognized as providers of medical eye care.[23]

This is a big step forward. Creating a cultural mind-set that includes an accurate understanding of what vision is and how it impacts learning and behavior is the next.

How do we want to spend our resources?

Some question the rehabilitative potential of older children and even adults with long-standing vision deficits. Dr. Susan Barry, a professor of neurobiology at Mount Holyoke College, has definitively provided an answer to this question in a very personal way. She developed strabismus in early infancy. Several surgeries corrected the cross-eyed positioning of her eyes; however, she was not able to see in three dimensions. This is called being stereoblind.

Without stereoscopy, there is an inability to see depth and judge distance. Space for her was compressed, and she had difficulties learning to read and drive. As a scientist she wondered about the malleability of the adult brain and whether she could correct her vision to perceive the world in 3-D. The common scientific belief had been that the brain was only capable of rewiring itself during a critical period in early childhood.

Her story, as told with touching candor in her book *Fixing My Gaze*, shares her journey as a young girl who dreaded school because reading was so difficult, to her discovery in college that she had been struggling with vision her whole life but did not know it. Curious, she began to ask questions and sought out research on vision.

Her inquisitiveness and persistence led to her discovery of behavioral optometry and vision therapy. By this time she was an accomplished college professor, and she took on her own vision challenges as a research study. Teaming with developmental optometrist Dr. Theresa Ruggiero, she persevered through a vision therapy program and emerged triumphant.

Dr. Oliver Sacks first shared her remarkable story with us in 2006 in his article "Stereo Sue," published in the *New Yorker* magazine. Her account of what it felt like to experience her first snowfall with her newfound ability to see in 3-D is extraordinarily moving.

Sue Barry verified that neuroplasticity is attainable beyond the flexible years of childhood and, what's more, influenced the principal beliefs of science by demonstrating the possibilities of brain development, adaptation, and rehabilitation. This holds tremendous promise and potential for future applications and study. Ironically, a team of doctors, optometrists, and developmental psychologists were collaborating at the Gesell Institute, right near the hospital where Sue was enduring surgery as a child. What was the focus of their work? It was none other than the study and treatment of cross-eyed children.

At that time, not unlike the present day, there was little cooperation and intercollegial support between eye surgeons and optometrists. For this reason, news of the leading-edge work at Gesell never reached Sue's parents. It took decades for Sue to finally benefit from vision therapy. There had existed the very real possibility that she never would have learned about it. Thankfully, her curiosity and unwavering determination did indeed result in an extraordinary difference in her own life, while bringing about the makings of possibility and hope for many, no matter what their age.[24]

Then there are those whose vision deficits get picked up because, uncommonly, the right pieces are present and aligned to offer an answer to their struggles. Sometimes, a persistent, mission-driven parent is one of those pieces.

Meet Jillian and Robin Benoit. Jillian was diagnosed with amblyopia when she was five years old. The road leading up to the discovery that she had been legally blind in one eye since birth was winding and complex. Her mom, Robin, can tell you what it's like firsthand to be a mom on a mission seeking help for her child. In fact, she did. Twice.

Jillian's Story: How Vision Therapy Changed My Daughter's Life is Robin's account of their six-year journey, from the initial first stages of worry, confusion, and uncertainty to the life-changing discovery of vision therapy. *Dear Jillian: Vision Therapy Changed My Life Too* is Robin's second literary gift to us, born of the overwhelming response of support and gratitude from readers worldwide. This book shares personal stories of children and adults who met with success and whose lives were forever changed for the better because of vision therapy.[25]

It's wonderful when individuals find their way and meet with success. With universal awareness, however, this is achievable for every child. Recognition and attention will no longer be left up to chance. This is especially significant when lack of information, resources, or support is the chief cause for inattention.

In an effort to rectify this, in April of 2001, Harvard University Graduate School of Education sponsored a conference on vision and learning titled "How Vision Impacts Literacy: An Educational Problem That Can Be Solved." This landmark occasion brought together behavioral optometrists and educational policy scholars to bridge the divide and collectively explore the connection between vision and learning.

A panel of optometrists presented their specialized findings to a captivated audience of educators and administrators. The issues included the limitations of school-based vision screenings, the high percentage of vision problems in poverty-stricken populations, the correlation between unrecognized vision problems and juvenile delinquency and illiteracy, and efforts to verify the efficacy of vision therapy as a successful method of treatment.

The outcome of the ensuing discussion led to this question: "How much will this cost and what is the expected return on investment?" The beauty of this forum created at Harvard rested in the intersection of fields represented. Doctors, educators, school leaders, and policy experts shared a roundtable opportunity to step across their respective peripheries, stand back, and examine the big picture. Each had the chance to learn about the challenges in other territories, leading to the big takeaway: collaboration is key to forward progress.

The Kansas Project, a research study implemented in 1993, was presented at the conference as a model for systematic change. Years of accumulated evidence of the link between vision and learning led to organized lobbying of the legislature by the Kansas Optometric Association. The resulting program, *See to Learn*, provided free vision screenings to preschoolers in optometric offices statewide. Additionally, the Kansas legislature approved funding for vision therapy to students presenting with vergence and accommodative disorders. In addition to providing essential eye care for children, this project will enable researchers to gather findings representative of the population, which will assist in future policy and planning decisions.

Dr. Rochelle Mozlin, a behavioral optometrist and associate professor at SUNY State College of Optometry and conference attendee, reported on the gathering in the *Journal of Behavioral Optometry*. In reflecting on the Kansas Project, she writes, "It is important to realize that this grant did not result from the work of one individual with expertise in the design of clinical trials. Rather, it grew from the collaborative efforts of dedicated practitioners across the state, who took small steps, baby steps forward, and built on each success. Now we are witnessing the snowball."[26]

Kentucky became the first state in the nation to legally require all children to undergo a comprehensive vision examination before entering school. This type of exam includes:

- complete general health and developmental history
- visual acuity measurement for closeup and distance
- measurement of refractive errors—nearsightedness, farsighted-ness, and astigmatism
- assessment of eye focusing, eye teaming, accommodation, ocular motility, and binocular vision skills
- examination of eye health

Several states are following their lead, including Massachusetts, Connecticut, and Missouri. None of these states is going it alone. Support for this advancement in policy and practical implementation comes from the American Optometric Association, the College of Optometrists in Vision Development, the American Academy of Optometry, the Optometric Extension Program Foundation, and Operation Bright Start (American Foundation for Vision Awareness).

Indeed, it took the team effort of doctors and researchers in concert with lawmakers to get the ball rolling. The goal behind the Kansas Project was to take a step beyond each individual doctor's threshold and create a mechanism for widespread attention and treatment. Dr. Mozlin brought further perspective to this action by underscoring the limitations for families due to the fact that all too often, insurance won't cover vision therapy. This deems it necessary for doctors to use a fee-for-service model, which in turn makes their services unattainable for some families. She points out with great clarity that, in order for policymakers to understand the connection between vision and learning, "there must be a shift toward a public health perspective."[27]

This is *key*.

The broad understanding of the importance of vision to a child's overall health blazed a new trail in the community of Framingham, Massachusetts. It began with school nurse Kathy Majzoub's observation that over the course of several years, the same children were identified with visual deficits in annual school screenings. Yet despite notifying the families of these children each time their vision evaluation rolled around, no follow-up occurred and the child was left untreated and at a disadvantage. The reasons for the lack of follow-up varied. Nonetheless, a frustrated school nurse felt compelled to step in and try to remedy the situation for these children.

She was successful in obtaining grant money to subsidize the cost of eyeglasses for those children who needed them. This was a big accomplishment, and the first of many steps she took to kick things into high gear. She opened a dialogue with Dr. Stacy Lyons, a pediatric optometrist at the New England College of Optometry. She shared her account with Dr. Lyons, who then brought her colleagues into the conversation. When asked what she would need to further help kids get their vision needs met, she replied, "A vision clinic in school."

That was eleven years ago, and today the Framingham Public Schools Vision Center is a tremendous asset to the school community, launched by the team effort of those on the front lines who "got it"— that vision is essential to a child's overall health, well-being, and success. Born of forward-thinking action, it is a model program for every community, everywhere.

This gives us pause to think about how many don't receive this specialized help in their lives and the losses incurred as a result. We know how it plays out for a child. Furthermore, in this increasingly unsustainable era of extreme expenditures, it stands to reason that investing our dollars in proactive objectives will ultimately be more cost-effective. There is a choice, along with great hope. It is important to realize that inaction is also a choice, and with this choice comes an undeniable cost.

Now equipped with this knowledge, let's choose wisely for our children, and for all of us.

7

THEIR FUTURE, OUR FUTURE

"**O**f the three-million nerve impulses that travel to the brain each second, two-thirds are generated from the eye. Approximately 70% of the sensory nerve fibers in the entire body originate from the eyes. From these statistics we can begin to understand the profound importance of vision as a process affecting development of the child and the learning process," writes Dr. William Padula, who practices neuro-visual processing rehabilitation and is a researcher in Connecticut.[1]

Dr. Padula's work is opening doors to a profoundly deeper understanding of the visual process and its relationship with the rest of the body, paving the way to an exciting future of broader treatment options and methods.

This substantiates the assertion made by Arnold Gesell, PhD, MD, a psychologist and pediatrician, who stated that "no organ focuses more concentrated energies," referring to the eyes.[2]

These are mind-bending pieces of information.

Everyone everywhere needs to understand what vision really is and why it is so deserving of attention and protection.

Protection? Indeed, Dr. Gesell said it rather prophetically more than half a century ago, during his time as director of the Yale University Clinic of Child Development.[3]

More accurately, he alluded to this idea in the form of a question: "Do we need a broader kind of visual hygiene to protect the growing eyes of today and tomorrow?"[4] Visual hygiene suggests following certain behaviors in the interest of protecting the eyes. Wearing sunglasses outdoors and protective eyewear when playing sports, using good lighting when reading, and limiting screen time are a few of the basics we can call out right off the bat. What his thought suggested, though, goes beyond these everyday sensible actions. Arnold Gesell was referring to a vision for the future.

Welcome to the future.

Now that we understand how vision is so central to learning, we must collectively acknowledge the magnitude of this awareness and focus attention on redesigning learning environments to support development symbiotically. This measure alone will transform education. It will do so first and foremost by transforming individual lives and then in part by reaping the returns from the contributions that well-educated, well-supported, and simply *well* children will make upon their assimilation into society.

To appreciate the relationship that education has with the overall nature of civilization, one must take a step back and look at all the parts involved in the whole. Just what, expressly, is the primary nucleus of the whole? It is the individual human being. Each life is precious. The use of the word *nature* in the opening sentence of this paragraph was chosen with careful intention. The *natural* aspect of living must be our starting point as we focus our thoughts on the direction in which education is heading.

Our connection with the natural world is so integral and fundamental to the human experience that once we stand back and look at the whole as well as our part in this whole, we begin to see the magnificent concept of interdependence at its finest. Yet we have lost touch with the natural rhythms that used to guide how we interact with time, space, and place—three key elements of our existence that now have no bounds.

We hold conversations on our cell phones while trying to converse with the person next to us, resulting in communication that lacks integrity and, in the latter case, eye contact. We bring our work home with us—to the dinner table, to our children's soccer games and dance recitals, even to our beds. The energy consumption alone necessary to maintain this 24/7 accessibility to everything and everyone is suspected to be harming individual and planetary health in ways we don't yet fully understand.

"Life is being designed so we don't have to use our eyes. We don't use our eyes nearly as much as we used to. Our culture of 'let's make things easier for ourselves' is making things infinitely harder for our children," asserts Joye Newman.

Technology has opened new doors to unimaginable advances, including the saving of countless lives, but we have to teach our children, and ourselves, how to use it wisely. The word *technology* likely conjures up a picture of an iPhone or a tablet in your mind's eye. Take it back a step. Picture, if you will, a lightbulb.

Before this invention in the 1800s, we used to arrange our lives and activities, including sleep, around the existing light from the sun. When it grew dark outside, we would wind down and go to sleep. Other than the warm glow from a lantern, we didn't have artificial lights or screens to rob our attention away from what our bodies naturally needed at the end of the day.

What's more, we felt this pull because we weren't distracted and tuned out from ourselves. Our behavior was in sync with the rising and setting of the sun and with the magnificent cycle of the seasons. This symbiotic relationship with naturally occurring phenomena is mirrored in the innate circadian rhythm that governs our sleep cycles. In effect, we have our own "rising and setting" timetable built into our bodies that is compatible with an astronomical agenda.

Current scientific research is investigating the potentially harmful effects of excessive exposure to light. The extended period of time in which we are exposed to it is one aspect; how it disturbs our sleep cycles and detracts from the quality of our sleep is another. Our inventions enable us to manipulate our environment and, we think, manage more while increasing our efficiency. But what are the costs, and are they worth it? In the interest of common sense, are we perchance moving far enough along down this path to be able to manage a healthy dose of hindsight?[5]

We know that a species becomes endangered when some other power decides that the natural resources inherent to its survival are expendable, such as land, water, and habitat. We also know that our actions as a species are endangering the lives of other creatures with whom we share this planet. We need to be concerned about how we choose to use our power to make decisions about human existence. In many ways, our culture has decided that the essentials for a healthy life are expendable, too. In actuality, we are endangering our own species.

In order to meet the demands in our professional lives so that we can earn income to sustain ourselves, we are often forced to take shortcuts and sacrifice sleep, exercise, and healthy eating habits because there just isn't enough time in the day to take the measures necessary to support these behaviors. While we are busy doing this, our children are sweating it out trying to meet the high-pressure demands they are encountering every day in school, so they can grow up and do the very same.

The home front is foundational to society. Its inherent stability, strength, and healthiness are largely dependent on the health of the individual or individuals who constitute it. Likewise, the health of communities is dependent on the health and stability of families. The needs of families, though, have become increasingly less important as society endeavors to compete in a world that has placed more value on what we achieve than what is necessarily good for us as human beings.

Consequently, we are seeing both physical and mental health suffer and conditions like obesity, diabetes, and depression increase because the basics are not given the importance they deserve. Our current model for living does not reflect wellness and balance, and we are all caught up in it. But our children are losing the most—their childhood. They are being overworked because school demands it, in turn because society demands it—so that they will do well on tests, so the government sees that they are "learning," so they can get into a good college, so they can get a good job, so they can join a society that values getting ahead despite the detriment to our personal well-being.[6]

The irony of all of this is we will burn kids out before they get the chance to grow up and lead the harried lives of their parents and bring up the next generation under the same unbalanced conditions, perpetuating the cycle. All to what end? In the rush to get to wherever we think we should be going, it is adding up to the degradation of our bodies, the planet, our lives, and our spirits. Whereas turning the tide toward a saner way of life may be a hard sell for some adults, we can no longer turn a blind eye toward the harm that is being imposed on our children. They depend on us. We need to step back and take a sobering look at how we got here.

The history and evolution of education are at once fascinating and concerning. How schools came to be the places they are today is a complex subject in and of itself. In our need to chart a sensible and reliable course going forward, looking back can afford us helpful, much-needed perspective. Interestingly, and ironically, when we look back we learn how much of our outlook was actually governed by looking forward, toward the future.

"A focus on the future dominates every aspect of children's lives. In education, an intense anxiety about the future has driven the standards movement," writes Dr. William Crain, a developmental psychologist who has studied this idea through a developmental lens throughout his career. In his highly acclaimed book, *Reclaiming Childhood*, he navigates the bumpy terrain of today's testing culture with a reliable map based on solid developmental truths. He explores at length how standardized testing is having a negative impact on students, pointing out that they are burdened by the academic demands and feeling the physical effects of stress, including headaches and sleep loss.[7]

The title page of the February 8, 2015, *New York Times Education Life* reads "Is Your First Grader College Ready?" flanked by a picture of a six-year-old holding up a hand-drawn, colored-by-crayon banner for North Carolina State. This is evidence of a growing belief that exposure to the concept of higher education at a very young age will motivate children to want to work harder so they will do well in school, and therefore go on to college. This mind-boggling mind-set is resulting in college tour field trips in fifth grade and discussions about dormitories in first grade.

"Young children simply cannot understand what college is," explained Dr. Marcy Guddemi, when interviewed for the article. "We are robbing children of childhood by talking about college and career so early in life."[8]

The rationale behind the standards movement is to set goals for our children's academic achievement with the presumption that this will ensure their success in the "real" world. However, this view takes the focus off children's developmental needs. In truth, to attain set goals, they must process through the stages of growth at the appropriate time so they are equipped and able to meet the progressive requisite skill requirements.

This controlled slant also interferes with a child's natural inclinations and inborn interests. Kids have a spark within them that, when fanned with encouragement, can allow them to find out what they are passionate about and what they are good at. It is our job to champion them on and support children in their quest to find out who they are meant to be and discover what they will contribute to the world as they mature.[9]

If you've ever sat and watched a child at play, you will notice that children exhibit an affinity for certain activities and enterprises from a very young age. We sometimes impose our agenda on our kids in the interest of exposing them to everything, with the well-intentioned hope of sharing all the world has to offer. This, we believe, will make them well rounded. But we have to realize that we can easily overwhelm them and inadvertently make the joyful and spontaneous act of discovery feel like a chore.

Children need the gifts of time and space so they can bloom. Gesell concluded that an inborn natural growth process is at work in human beings, and when endowed with the freedom and the right conditions, we flourish.[10]

Likening the progression of a child's maturation to the building of a house, William Crain points out that the integrity of the finished structure will only be as strong as the stability of the foundation. He validates parents' concerns about their children's future success but reassures us that allowing them to fully experience the precious time that is childhood in full measure will prepare them to meet their future equipped and whole.

"We serve the future by protecting the present," affirms Maria Montessori.[11]

We can reflect at this juncture and see where these movements have brought us. In rewinding the tape, we revisit several initiatives that were at the forefront of major changes in viewpoint and position on how education was lacking in this country, where it should be going, and what its overarching objectives should be. Prior to this new era of questions and alarm, teachers had much more autonomy and freedom in their classrooms. With the arrival of painstaking inquiry into declining test scores, widespread illiteracy, and written language deficiencies, things began to change.

In April of 1983, President Ronald Reagan presented the country with the thirty-six-page report *A Nation At Risk* and declared America's

schools inferior and glaringly inadequate. The report summoned re-
forms to stem the tide that the direction our schools were headed in,
which, as the title of the report bluntly indicated, was putting "our
nation at risk." Specifically, actions were urged on several fronts, including the creation of learning standards, a more rigorous curriculum,
extending the length of the school day and the school year, and more
competitive teachers' salaries to help increase teacher retention. [12]

For all intents and purposes, this report launched the school reform
movement, referred to more commonly today with strong emotion as
the standards movement.

More than thirty years later, and with an increase in expenditure that
is more than double what it was in the 1980s, little has improved. Test
scores have barely moved, teacher salaries have improved minimally,
and student achievement remains static. Concerns that we were not
sufficiently preparing students for the future, which would compromise
our country's pace in the global economy, were echoed in similar re-
ports that came out in the decades that followed.

No Child Left Behind (NCLB), put forth by President George W.
Bush in January 2001 three days after he took office, attempted to level
the playing field so all children can reach proficiency. This law encompasses five principles: Standards and Assessment, Accountability and
Early Years Progress, Corrective Action, Staff Qualifications, and Parental Involvement. [13]

In attempting to level the playing field, however, this program has in
actuality created chaotic divergence. It put into place rigorous compli-
ances, consequences for teachers and entire school districts, and the
built-in option for parents to choose to send their child to another
school within the district that shows higher performance ratings. The
focus on authentic teaching and learning grew dim. The confusion and
the pressure were discouraging to teachers and served to make their
jobs markedly more difficult. Most importantly, all these boundaries
and courses of action circumvented what education really needed to
help kids achieve.

As of this writing, there has come about a bipartisan effort to revise
NCLB. These proposed changes would allow individual states to choose
how to remedy schools that are struggling and create their own teacher
evaluation protocols. Washington would no longer have a blanket say in
matters. The numbers of tests kids have to take would still remain the

same, at least for now, but they would hold less weight. Teacher assessment would not be tied to student test scores, which would relieve them of much unfair pressure. Additionally, schools would no longer be penalized by the federal government if they fail to reach the set benchmarks. Overall, these changes are being seen as much more equitable. And while discussion and debate will ensue within the walls of Congress as this process unfolds, it is encouraging to witness recognition and dialogue about these critical issues. [14]

In more recent years, we have been witness to President Obama's *Race to the Top* (RTTT) initiative. RTTT is an incentive-based competitive grant program that rewards districts and states with heavy sums of money in recognition of substantial improvements in student success. Individual states must apply for these funds. The four areas of attention include:

- adopting standards and assessments that prepare students to succeed in college and the workplace and to compete in the global economy;
- building data systems that measure student growth and success and that inform teachers and principals about how they can improve instruction;
- recruiting, developing, rewarding, and retaining effective teachers and principals, especially where they are needed most;
- turning around the lowest-achieving schools. [15]

Analysis by the *Broader Bolder Approach to Education* campaign indicates that there exist some imbalances with this effort. In short, limitations of time and resources and holes in the strategic fabric put into place to address the achievement gap have limited the attainability of the anticipated gains of this program. Here we see the issue of sustainability surfacing, as so many moving parts make managing steps toward change unwieldy and precarious. [16]

Note that with the current discussion in Congress regarding NCLB, there is still substantial forward movement that needs to occur beyond these anticipated positive changes. We've taken so many steps backward over time that these policy improvements bring us back roughly to where we started. So while we think we're in a better position, we are actually in a "less worse" position. We are still facing the same problems that have eluded answers for too long.

Could it be that these initiatives are asking the wrong questions and putting the wrong concerns under the microscope? What if we focused on the inborn developmental needs of the child? Would answers to the hot topics that have plagued education begin to fall into place with the right methodology guiding our decisions and policies? Some will allege this is an overly simplistic or naïve stance. In spite of this, a case could be made for shaping enriching, accommodating foundational learning experiences that would likely reduce the degree of need for intervention that we are witnessing today.

In an ideal world, we would be asking the question, "What is in the best interest of the child?" In an ideal world, we would be responding to this essential question with reliable answers and supporting them with appropriate actions. We know the answers. Decades of findings by top researchers in child development have spelled them out for us. The sound, time-tested research findings of Gesell are looked upon as some of the most reliable and respected criterion. He is considered by many to be the father of the field of child development. "Dr. Gesell was the first to study the ages and stages of development," states Dr. Marcy Guddemi.[17]

"Indeed," writes Gesell in his classic text *Vision: Its Development in Infant and Child*, "vision is so intimately identified with the whole child that we can not understand its economy and its hygiene without investigating the whole child." His insight into vision's role in the development of the whole child fostered many insightful questions and inspired in-depth research spanning decades. His perception afforded his peers a perspective view of where we were in our scope of understanding, as well as where we needed to go.

Noting that a substantial degree of knowledge existed about the eye as an organ, much of the information we had accumulated stemmed from studies on adults. This mostly dealt with the eye's mechanics, physiology, and visual efficiency. Gesell astutely pointed out that we understood little about the origins of visual function and how this characteristic develops as the child matures. He was apt to point out that we could no longer work under the assumption that the eyes of a child process the world in the same manner as the eyes of an adult.

Through unparalleled quantifiable research, Gesell was able to ascertain that visual development is a rapid process that, while subtle in its evolution, is deducible to the attentive observer. Beginning in infancy, visual development shows indications of interaction with motor development and coordination. The eyes lead the movement of the hands as they reach out to touch and manipulate objects, and the hands, at times, lead the eyes when they gaze at that which is within their grasp.

Successive studies of preschool and school-aged children contributed a rich cross-section analysis of general sequential behavior. The expansive study of whole child development at Yale was a comprehensive endeavor comprising four areas of specialized focus: motor behavior, adaptive behavior, language behavior, and personal-social behavior. Throughout cumulative inquiry, distinct studies of visual behavior grew from these in quantity and significance. It became clear that vision played an active role in all four areas of concentrated study listed above.

Of particular importance is the recognition that vision is highly engaged with movement and the motor systems of the body. Gesell regarded them as "inseparable." How visual development progresses in a child is largely an expression of the hardwired embryonic schematic that governs this unfolding process throughout maturation. This includes what Gesell calls the "action system," referring to the natural progression of movement and coordination. In the nature versus nurture discussion, we can think of this as the "nature" piece.

As children's motor abilities increase and they adapt to their spatial surroundings, take on more activity, and increase their extent of exploration, the interplay between their physical stature and the structure of their environment will be a factor in their developing physical posture. This is a key influential ingredient in determining the course of their visual development. This is where the "nurture" piece plays into the picture. [18]

We take for granted a plain fact that Gesell paid much attention to—we are continually adjusting our bodily position in space to counter the constant pull of gravity. Posture is a key aspect of visual function. The highly intricate configurations of muscle groupings throughout the entire body have evolved ingeniously to work in concert and support movement as well as sensory processing. In addition to the more obvious larger muscles, even the smallest muscles of the eyes play into the manifestation of a person's posture. [19]

The question often arises regarding how we know scientifically what a child sees, especially at such young ages. Gesell identified the progression of neuromotor behavior patterns in utero by studying images obtained using cinemamicrophotographic techniques by fellow researchers. These observations established a knowledge base of the physiological actions exhibited during development. He and his team were then able to formulate an understanding of how these responses integrate to respond to and with movement and perception.

The sophisticated learning Gesell's research team acquired from here derived from intensive observation of the actions of children at all stages of development. Changes and evolution of movement patterns and adaptations of the body reflected the very same events occurring in the visual system. Gesell explains, "The eyes are always in the total behavior picture. At any given moment, either they are directing the postural set of the entire organism, or they are registering the effect of local and general postural sets."

In other words, the processing of information coming into the brain through the visual system has a direct affect on how one perceives and maneuvers one's body and actions in relation to one's spatial context. Likewise, how a person interacts with his or her surroundings will greatly impact that person's visual perception and functioning.[20]

The last chapter of Gesell's *Vision: Its Development in Infant and Child* is appropriately titled "The Conservation of Child Vision." It was with great foresight that he brought to light the extensive implications of visual hygiene on society. He delineated then the need for collaboration among parents, educators, pediatricians, lawmakers, and lay leaders to ensure the well-being of children as they grow up. He urged that children's visual development be evaluated and managed from the early years on through adulthood.

Calling the need for visual care a "ubiquitous problem" due to its importance and justifiable need for committed attention, Gesell's words again rang prophetically when he stated, "It involves the public, as well as the professions, and it requires a policy of continuous general education as to the psychological meaning of sight and the far-reaching implications of visual health." He also underscored the need for cooperation between professions and urged this on.[21]

Today the Gesell Institute carries on the extraordinary work of Arnold Gesell by supporting the healthy development of children through parent and teacher education workshops, professional development, and the dissemination of informational tools and publications. Guidelines for instruction, teaching practices, and development of curricula offer educators sound advice when designing learning environments. Parents have access to current research-based materials that illuminate the developmental stages through which children progress, enabling them to support their child at home and in partnership with their school.[22]

Gesell's theory of child development is identified as "a maturational-developmental theory." It documented phases of growth that were originally published in 1925 as the *Gesell Developmental Schedules.* His research findings specify that all children progress through natural, inborn stages of development that have a set sequential path. While all children move through these stages as they grow, they don't all do so at the same pace.

So reliable and accurate were his findings, they have stood the test of time and remain a respected, trustworthy guide for understanding developmental behavior in children. Psychologists, pediatricians, and child development specialists turn to his teachings to guide them in caring for children. It is common to see Gesell and his work referenced in wide pools of literature on child development.

"The child is more than a score," declared Arnold Gesell. These words ring in our minds today in ways he probably could not even have imagined. If we push our kids to take on tasks before they are developmentally ready, the need for special services to fix the damage later on will only increase. This is already occurring, and many would argue that it has been the case for a long time.

Thinking back to chapter 5, where we discussed the inundation experienced by child study teams, we need to understand that this need could possibly increase even more over time. For example, we don't fully know how our screen culture will affect development. The Kaiser Family Foundation Study in January 2010, titled *Generation M²: Media in the Lives of 8- To 18-Year-Olds*, examined the quantity and quality of media use in children in America. Their findings, which were staggering, showed that kids spend between nine and eleven hours with media a day.

The current high-pressure, test-and-standards-driven academic culture is adding jet fuel to an already imbalanced model of education. In truth, learning conditions have become extreme, and we cannot yet even fully perceive of the consequences.

The consequences, though, are likely to have a far-reaching ripple effect. In truth, they already are, and this is factoring into why education has grown to be so unsustainable for everyone involved—students, teachers, families, whole communities, and the entire nation. More than this, deep concerns lie with regard to how our children are going to manage their lives once out in the world. They are struggling to manage them now in the face of enormous overload.

These issues inspired Wall Street lawyer turned filmmaker Vicki Abeles to take serious action when she began to notice the effects of the high-pressure academic culture impacting her own family and community. Deeply concerned, moved by a sense of urgency, and motivated to document the individual stories that were playing out among school-age children, she pursued her own inquiry into the issues and created a film that has been viewed nation-wide by more than one million people and counting.

If you haven't seen *Race to Nowhere*, please find your way to a screening.

The goal of this film is to boldly place children's well-being center stage, in the spotlight, and bring an unprecedented level of attention to the school-related stressors that are wreaking havoc with our children's mental and physical health. Interviews with students, parents, teachers, pediatricians, psychologists, college professors, and education advocates revealed very difficult truths about how life really is for students today. Given a voice and the opportunity to share their stories, those whom Abeles spoke with disclosed heartrending experiences resulting from the demands placed on them by school.

Changes to homework policies, academic course load, testing procedures, college preparation, and school schedules are now being examined through a healthier lens by many communities to help restore balance to education and the lives of kids and their families. The sweeping effect that this film has had since its release indicates that it most definitely hit a nerve for the masses. Recognizing the immeasurable value of succeeding in areas of life that are not typically part of a school curriculum, *Race to Nowhere* has heroically declared *valid* all the truly important facets of childhood and growing up.[23]

It seems we are individually and collectively hitting the pause button and stopping to look at where we are. Maybe due to desperation, or just sheer exhaustion, whatever the cause it is a very good step. The real question is, what is keeping us from acting on the ideal mentioned earlier?

This ideal is not some far-fetched, fantasy-laden idea without base in reality. We have the expertise, skills, and talent to respond with brilliance to what is in the best interest of children. Our educational system needs to honor the developmental stages that children progress through, which means a radical shift from what we are used to and currently experiencing. Today's kids are attending school in what may be the most pressure-filled, stress-inducing environment since the start of formal education.

There is something very wrong with our learning model if we have to medicate children to stay afloat within it. Certainly, we want our kids to do better than simply staying afloat. We want them to be able to swim.

We can turn this ship around. It's an enormous ship, and the global current is strong, but there is strength in many minds, hearts, and hands coming together, and momentum can be shifted. Beyond determination and drive, we have a growing scientific knowledge base verifying linkage between environmental influences and learning outcomes. We are equipped to do this.

8

A VISION FOR LEARNING

There is an abundance of ongoing discussion about how children should learn and how teachers should teach. Really, though, when it comes to learning, there is no justification for "shoulds." One cannot force a child to learn.

"We can only create an environment that encourages and motivates learning," points out Dr. Linda Tamm. "We can create or recreate an opportunity for curiosity and confidence that facilitates knowledge and problem solving, and we can create a context that encourages development, like a seed in good soil. But telling a seed it must grow is not going to make it so!" she elucidates.

Excellent metaphor.

Children learn in different ways. An overview of one position describes the presence of visual, auditory, and kinesthetic modalities through which a child processes information via sensory input. Visual learners have a propensity for learning through seeing, auditory learners through listening, and kinesthetic learners through movement, touch, and active "doing." The thinking is that children may favor one of these areas but can also demonstrate a combination of two or even all three in varying degrees. [1]

How children process and express learned knowledge is as unique as their fingerprints. An endless combination of variables will impact how this occurs, and it is a lifelong, fluid process. Yet we have identified patterns and archetypes, leading to theories and methodologies that attempt to reach all learners. One key to accomplishing this is to create learning environments that are logistically able to function as a whole, while allowing room for individuality and creativity to thrive.

This requires the science of best practices, but just as children have their own unique ways of learning, teachers have their own unique ways of teaching. Facilitating the blending of both of these pieces is what makes teaching an art.

The theory of multiple intelligences was originated by Dr. Howard Gardner, a world-renowned psychologist and professor of cognition and education at Harvard University Graduate School of Education. His theory has received a tremendous amount of attention since its inception just over thirty years ago. Based on his interdisciplinary research regarding how human capabilities present in the brain, he postulates that we all have a unique variety of abilities that function, to a certain extent, independent of one another. This is in contrast to the view that we possess one mode of intelligence that impacts how we fare across the board.[2]

THE EIGHT TYPES OF MULTIPLE INTELLIGENCES
HOWARD GARDNER, PHD, HARVARD UNIVERSITY

Verbal/Linguistic Intelligence—"Word Smart"

Learners with this strength are able to:

- Think in words
- Use spoken and written language effectively to express themselves
- Understand the order and meaning of words
- Remember words and their definitions easily
- Use language to express and appreciate complex meanings

Logical/Mathematical Intelligence—"Number/Reasoning Smart"

Learners with this strength are able to:

- Analyze problems logically and use deductive thinking patterns
- Calculate and carry out complete mathematical operations
- Excel at complex mathematical calculations
- Recognize and understand abstract patterns
- Perceive relationships and connections
- Use abstract, symbolic thought and deductive reasoning

Spatial Intelligence—"Picture Smart"

Learners with this strength are able to:

- Think in three dimensions
- Recognize, use, and interpret images and patterns
- Reproduce objects in three dimensions
- Understand and recognize relationships between objects
- Possess a strong imagination

Musical Intelligence—"Music Smart"

Learners with this strength are able to:

- Perform, compose, and appreciate musical patterns
- Understand the structure of music with a natural inclination
- Attune themselves to sounds and rhythms
- Recognize change in pitch, tone, rhythm, and timbre
- Apply mathematical thinking patterns to music, which often overlap

Bodily/Kinesthetic Intelligence—"Body Smart"

Learners with this strength are able to:

- Use the body for expression
- Manipulate objects and use a variety of physical skills
- Expertly control movement and coordination—fine-motor or gross-motor or both
- Naturally incorporate a sense of timing

- Find it easy to connect the mind with the body

Naturalist Intelligence—"Nature Smart"

Learners with this strength are able to:

- Recognize and appreciate relationships in the natural world
- Discriminate among living things—plants and animals
- Be sensitive to features of the natural world
- Possess a deep understanding and respect for nature

Interpersonal Intelligence—"People Smart"

Learners with this strength are able to:

- See things from the perspectives of others easily
- Communicate well verbally and nonverbally
- Work well with others
- Understand people's intentions, motivations, and desires
- Be sensitive to the moods and temperaments of others
- Create and maintain healthy relationships

Intrapersonal Intelligence—"Self Smart"

Learners with this strength are able to:

- Understand themselves
- Understand their "self" in relation to others
- Be aware of and capable of expressing their feelings
- Interpret and appreciate their own thoughts and motivations and use this knowledge in planning their lives
- Appreciate the *self* and also the human condition

So influential has this concept been, it has spawned a genesis of entire schools and curricula fashioned in this theory all over the world. It has become an area of study unto itself, and Gardner's work has taken a place alongside that of some of the most influential thinkers in history.[3]

A forward-thinking vision emerged from Gardner's distinguished analysis of schools, society, and human intellect decades ago. Recognizing that some critics considered then, as even now, child-centered education to be utopian, he proposed the following viewpoint: "To my mind, the real obstacles to individual-centered education are not financial constraints or knowledge limitations, but rather questions of will. So long as we choose to believe that the individual-centered approach is not valid, or, even if valid, simply not practical, it will appear utopian. If, however, we decide to embrace the goals and the methods of individual-centered education, I have no doubt that we can make significant progress in that direction," he states in *Multiple Intelligences: The Theory in Practice*.

To complement this position, he presents a paradigm for renewing education reform that is rooted in cooperation and collaboration. This model forms its basis in community, above all else. "In a viable community, members recognize their differences and strive to be tolerant, while learning to talk constructively with one another and perennially searching for common ground," Gardner affirms.

This community-focused model turns the discussion from an enforced, top-down direction to one in which "everyone has a voice." Acknowledging difficulty, challenges, and discomfort inherent to the process, Gardner reassures us that such growing pains are surmountable and must be endured to effectively engage in problem solving and forward progress. "Far from representing sentimental rhetoric, a commitment to community reveals a recognition of the hard realities required for effectiveness in today's world," he upholds.[4]

A child-centered approach to teaching and learning is a philosophy that would respectfully embrace the developmental needs of the whole child and allow for the child's unique strengths and aptitudes to take root. While there is debate about the feasibility and effectiveness of this approach, there is a great deal of rationale that supports its validity. Contesting pedagogical choices seems to be routine, a rite of passage even, as new administrations turn over in government and within the field of education itself.

Ask a teacher who has been teaching for more than ten years. That teacher will likely tell you that trends come and go. Former methods that were declared outdated or ineffective resurface in time with a shiny new label, though the ideology is the same or closely similar. Strategies get recycled and renamed and boomerang back to teachers, who must recalibrate their lesson plans and units of study. Routinely. This becomes an additional load on top of a teacher's already overloaded agenda of responsibilities. The technology factor complicates this. Navigating through fluctuating tactics of, say, delivering instruction and tracking assessment through a cyber approach consumes much time and energy, especially when the technology system itself changes so frequently.

The challenges kids are dealing with today raise the question—are we waking up to the detrimental effects of child-*uncentered* methodologies? With standards and testing protocols running the show more than ever before, parents and teachers are exasperated. So are kids. This is a topic of conversation that is dominating our consciousness, and concerns flow freely at soccer matches, scout meetings, and gatherings of all sorts. It is prompting new levels of questioning, doubt, and protest. The recent display of unprecedented parental pushback to the standardized testing regime is a glaring example.[5]

Education is a field deserving of the utmost support and respect. It is looked upon to contribute more and more to the greater whole, indeed even to *fix* the greater whole, while getting by with less and less. This is unfair to everyone and is a discrepancy that may actually be contributing to the many ills we struggle with as a society. But we need to compassionately wrap our minds around the idea that it can also be a resolution to them, if we heed the call.

It is unacceptable to exploit our youngest, most vulnerable citizens on a selfishly driven quest to be number one. In doing so, we remain blind to the truth—that we are actually creating a populace of depleted, ill-equipped, dispirited human beings who will be unprepared to contribute productively to the future of society and find personal fulfillment. While neglect of their basic human rights bears out more mutedly while they are young, innocent, and voiceless, the injurious consequences speak out loudly and in abundance as the effects begin to catch up with them.

What if we embraced a child-centered approach to educating our children that would resolutely place child development at the core of learning? In doing so, a child's growth would be supported as opposed to impeded. Of paramount importance is the role that vision plays in learning and overall development. This belongs on the map in a guiding capacity toward amending a refurbished ideology.

Gesell's understanding of vision was holistic—vision is part of the whole child. In the interest of supporting the healthy development of children's vision, as in the protective sense that Gesell suggested, balanced learning activities and appropriate skill requirements would be at the heart of curriculum design. The basis for this rationale lies in the well-substantiated central role that vision plays in the entirety of the processes that support learning. Since vision is pivotal to all areas of achievement, ensuring that this sensory area is given every opportunity to develop fully and unhampered should be a core focus for educators.

Liken this to physical education and we can identify a strong parallel. We acknowledge the importance of a fit body. We must also realize the importance of fit vision. Schools ideally should support physical fitness. Schools should also support visual fitness. Dr. Stacy Lyons accentuates the definition of wellness to include healthy, functioning vision. When a child can see clearly and process proficiently, success and accomplishment follow, leading to positive self-esteem and confidence. In contrast, when the opposite is true, the ill effects need no explanation.

Through such implementation, it is likely that we will reduce the prevalence of vision problems we are seeing in children. This model for an overall health-promoting learning environment would also include in-house resources to provide vision care to those children who need it. This would include vision therapy. VT belongs right alongside all the other support services that children receive, so that every child has the chance to reach his or her full potential.

"We know that eventually fuller visual coverage will be needed for all children than is now available," write Drs. Frances L. Ilg and Louise Bates Ames in their distinguished book *School Readiness: Behavior Tests Used at the Gesell Institute*. "Information obtained from Snellen Acuity charts barely scratches the surface and reveals only some of the gross difficulties. We do not consider it an adequate measure of a child's visual functioning. Schools need to know much more about vision than this test reveals."

"We know that visual experts need to be trained more fully in the principles of visual behavior and developmental vision. Though it may be some time before school systems will include a visual specialist as part of their regular staff, the service of such a specialist should be available to all school systems. All need to know more than most now do about the visual functioning of their pupils."[6]

Their words were first published in the mid 1960s. It's high time for knowledge about vision-related learning problems to become mainstream, so that policies can be created to foster implementation of programs that will address these problems that have long been hidden from view. Once this is achieved, we will likely see numbers of students in special education programs decrease when deficiencies will be correctly recognized and addressed.

In addition to making a case for this on a strong emotional level, the most practical way to effect positive change may be to do the math. Funds can be more efficiently and appropriately channeled toward resources that will support the recognition and treatment of vision problems. This is where the savings will occur. That is, recognizing and treating hidden vision disorders will save schools tens of thousands of dollars. With 25 percent of children affected by a vision problem that is impeding their ability to learn, many of these children wind up in special education programs. In some cases, children are shipped out of district to special schools, costing the district even more money for transportation. In other cases, children will drop out of school, costing society on many different levels.

Of course, since vision problems do more than impact children academically, these challenges can take an emotional toll and spiral into behavioral problems resulting from low self-esteem. Beyond needing help with learning as they struggle in school, children then also need support from guidance counselors, school social workers, and psychologists for emotional problems that are secondary symptoms. The need for these services to address these consequential problems is overflowing, feeding into a system unequipped to address this critical area. It is a vicious cycle.

Here we further build the case for comprehensive vision evaluations becoming *standard*. A joint study by Drs. Joel Zaba, Rochelle Mozlin, and William T. Reynolds compared the outcomes of vision screenings versus full vision examinations. Their findings bring to light striking concerns.

First, the limitations of vision screenings were clear. "Vision screenings certainly play an important role in identifying visual dysfunctions in a variety of settings. However, our data strongly indicates that, in the case of youngsters entering school for the first time, vision screenings can identify some youngsters with visual dysfunctions, but can miss a significant number of others."[7]

Compliance is another factor that greatly reduces the degree of help that vision screenings provide. While they are not the ideal, screenings will still identify students with acuity problems, amblyopia, and strabismus. Studies have shown that a significant percentage of children do not receive the recommended follow-up care.

A lack of communication with parents is one cause. One study showed that half of the parents of children who had failed a vision screening were made aware of this. In another it was found that, on average, four years went by between a failed vision screening and the child being taken to an eye doctor for a vision examination. A lot of complications can occur for a child during such a stretch of time, with regard to both vision and school success.

Now, keep in mind that this is fallout just from inconsistencies with vision screenings, which are inherently limited in their scope of detecting more hidden visual disorders. Getting back to the math, there is a price for the domino effect that results from untreated vision problems. The U.S. Department of Health and Human Services reported that, in 1995, the monetary impact of vision disorders and disabilities on the U.S. economy was more than $38.4 billion.[8]

The same report that has its sights set on current and future objectives as outlined in the "Healthy People 2020" program proposes a 10 percent increase in the number of preschool children who receive vision screenings, bringing the percentage from 40.1 percent to 44.1 percent. Developed by the U.S. Preventative Services Task Force, the screening aims to assess visual acuity and detect for amblyopia and related risk factors.[9]

It would stand to reason that the $38.4 billion price tag referenced above did not take into account the unidentified costs linked to children mistakenly classified or medicated due to an incorrect diagnosis. This reasoning is based on the observation that the "Healthy People" model only attends to visual acuity and amblyopia. If it factored in all the other vision disorders that affect children, the cost would be likely be radically different.

Children with vision problems that go undetected inevitably grow up to be adults with vision problems, and this reality is reflected in the literacy problem that compromises our workforce. Many of the conditions in today's workplace demand a high degree of skill, organization, and the ability to function efficiently in a fast-paced, ever-changing environment. Deficient literacy skills, it has been shown statistically, cost U.S. taxpayers and businesses billions of dollars in profits and productivity. In 2006, $5.9 billion was spent by U.S. organizations to teach basic skills such as remedial reading, writing, and math to employees. [10]

This potentially higher cost resulting from choosing not to invest resources in comprehensive vision evaluations over screenings should get communal attention.

> Economics are often used to justify vision screenings as the best system to reliably detect most vision problems at a much lower cost than providing vision examinations for all children. Certainly, if one considers only the direct costs of services, then a vision screening is far less expensive than a comprehensive vision examination. However, in order to be valid, all indirect as well as direct costs associated with each procedure must be included in the comparison. Given the large number of vision disorders that are missed by vision screenings, the indirect costs are likely substantial, if not incalculable. How can the negative impact of an undiagnosed vision problem on the academic performance and quality of life of these children be calculated? [11]

So much of the hard work has been done. We have the know-how and science to detect these disorders and treat them successfully. We know that doing so will improve individual and collective lives. In order for this to occur systemically so that all children who need help will get help, there are actions to be taken on educational policy and economic fronts. There are important answers and solutions to logistic challenges that need to be found.

This is achievable.

Dr. Brenda Montecalvo, a behavioral optometrist who lectures internationally, offers an insightful perspective on the measures needed to accommodate the developing vision needs of children. Of greatest importance is the need for a standard definition of what a comprehensive vision evaluation is, since it can mean different things to different practitioners. This will necessitate identifying what questions need to be asked and answered about a child's vision prior to entering school.

These questions need to be standard as well, so that all children are being screened properly and uniformly. These measures need to be mandated at the federal level.

She states that insurance companies need to understand what vision is and cover the ideal standardized comprehensive vision evaluation all kids need to undergo before entering school and then yearly. Insurance companies also need to be educated about the interrelationship that vision has with other behaviors and conditions. By covering VT, this may eliminate or reduce the need for other services down the road, some of which may require lengthy maintenance and greater costs in the long run.

Dr. Montecalvo points out that in order to have vision therapy available in schools alongside other services such as occupational therapy and speech therapy, it has to be available to everyone. She identifies two central challenges while exploring how to do this effectively.

The first is that vision therapy in schools may not ensure all the care that is needed for every child simply because there may not be the resources to support it. Due to time and staffing limitations, reaching every child with a need, and doing so to the degree necessary so that it's fully effective, is dependent on conditions that may be inconsistent. The second is that getting private care involves other challenges—parental follow-up, home regimen support, and cost and insurance coverage. These are also fluctuating variables.

The question is: Should vision therapy be systemized within our schools or remain privatized?

The answer is: it should be both.

With the exception of the few schools that have heeded the call and brought vision services on board within their districts, children's vision care is by and large handled privately. In either scenario, variations in the degree of care children get are a reality. This is of greater concern among families affected by poverty.

The findings of Dr. Charles Basch's study out of Columbia University fostered the following conclusion:

> Vision problems are highly and disproportionately prevalent among school-aged urban minority youth, have a negative impact on academic achievement through their effects on sensory perceptions, cognition, and school connectedness, and effective practices are available for schools to address these problems. School-based vision

screening programs are a logical approach for the early detection and treatment of vision problems affecting youth and are widely implemented in the nation's schools. To more fully realize the educational (and public health) benefits of current investments in screening, programs will require improved follow-up and coordination between and among agencies conducting screening, school nurses, teachers and parents, and in some cases community resources. [12]

One of the challenges in providing eye care for kids is making sure they receive the follow-up treatment they need. For children living in poverty and poor home conditions, this is a stumbling block. We provide education for all children, along with other services they may need, through the schools. Paying heed to the critical importance of vision and its effects bearing out in the life of a child, this is an area that must receive attention too. It is especially crucial for children who are living with disadvantages. [13]

Dr. Leonard Press holds the view that VT in schools is feasible, and that it should be a nationwide model. While the first question most often asked is how we will pay for it, this is not where his focus lies. Not because it isn't important, but because something else needs attention first. He conveys that we have to rectify the "simplistic, archaic view of what vision is," as he points out. Many still understand it to be only about eyesight. The world needs to become "vision literate."

To accomplish this, he explains, a logical means to this end would be through teacher training. The broader knowledge of what vision is and its relationship to learning must become common knowledge among educators. The research findings of Dr. Darell Harmon, as an example, receive little attention today. Our current circumstances are reason to pick up where he left off. This goal can be reached in two ways.

First, vision development must be taught in teacher education programs. Teaching teachers *why* vision matters is key. Higher education would be a portal to future implementation of vision support services for all children. Again, a standard is needed here to ensure that all student teachers are receiving the necessary information, much like they would when learning about other established areas of child development.

Second, for those already in the field, widespread professional development training would equip teachers with this knowledge. Creating such a curriculum that would provide continuing education for teachers is an essential, forward-thinking, and potential-laden concept. This is fertile ground for future study, as visual development is factored into learning design.

If you are a teacher reading this, no doubt the first thing that may have popped into your head involves the ever-mounting fear of more paperwork. Rightfully so. Documentation required by red tape rules and regulations is a full-time job in and of itself. This ties in with why we need to make education more sustainable, which includes the notion of how time is spent and on what. But if children will learn better, guided by developmentally appropriate signposts, it is likely that many of the hoops we have created and continue to re-create, to jump through to improve education, may no longer be needed.

Education needs a serious overhaul, and it should start with recognizing the function that vision has in how kids learn. "Vision development, its role in learning and behavior, and why it needs to be addressed with services in schools is critical, and this information needs to reach everyone," Dr. Press contends. "Whether we are talking about AD/HD, poor school performance, autism or concussions, we are still coming back to the same bottleneck because we're using an 1800s model of evaluating children for visual problems. As a result, they are going unrecognized and kids are falling through the cracks," he further emphasizes.

A working model we can turn to when envisioning vision therapy in schools is the field of occupational therapy (OT). Dr. Press, who works closely with many occupational therapists, puts it in perspective. Children who need and qualify for occupational therapy have the opportunity to receive this service in school because it is offered. While this is beneficial for students, it is providing a somewhat more limited extent of treatment given the confines of time and staff availability. Private consultation with occupational therapists would offer more in-depth rehabilitation, though at an additional cost.

Still, children receiving OT in school are certainly going to be helped to some degree and are better off than if they were not receiving any services at all. For those students whose need is minimal, school-based OT can be sufficient. In this same vein, vision services would be offering help to many students who might otherwise not get any. In Framingham, Massachusetts, for example, the school vision clinic is providing eyeglasses for students with acuity problems. "Plain old visual acuity is as much of a need," Dr. Stacy Lyons points out. Simple enough: when kids can't see clearly, they won't function well. The clinic provides complimentary exams, follow-up care, and eyeglasses paid for by grant money for those whose families can't afford them. Vision therapy services are also provided. Parents are encouraged to be present on-site to engage in the process with their children.

This model is replicable. The components necessary to launch such a program include:

- a community mind-set open to understanding what wellness actually means—and that vision is a part of this definition;
- school buy-in: board and committees, superintendent, principals, teachers, child study team, nurses, and support personnel;
- ongoing outreach education to community;
- logistics and funding.

If we explore the history of how OT came to be offered in schools, we can glean sharp insights about the multiple fronts that must come together to effect change and growth. And this is what happened in the United States in the early 1970s. A groundswell of activism promoting civil rights for individuals paid particular attention to children with disabilities.

Parents, teachers, and administrators lobbied at the federal level to advocate for children with disabilities to have equal access to educational opportunities that would meet their needs. In 1975, their efforts were recognized with the landmark passage of Public Law 94-142—the Education for All Handicapped Children Act. This historic legislative move reflected a shift in thinking about how our culture viewed education.

As societal values evolved, education came to be viewed as not only a system that teaches content, but also one that prepares students for learning. This was viewed as "a radical departure from the traditional view of the function of public education and established the need for inter-professional interaction."[14]

The concept of bringing OT into schools brought with it certain challenges that, in effect, can be thought of as growing pains. The creators of the law pointed out that in the rising commitment to attend to the "whole" child, individuals from different respective professions would need to adjust to a collaborative approach in the interest of meeting this overarching goal. Partnerships between specialists in the educational and medical professions would be crucial.

Through additional grassroots efforts and lobbying, the law was amended several times. In addition to serving the OT needs of school children ages five and up, the law entitles preschool children ages three to five to services to help get them ready for school. In addition, children from birth to two years are eligible for services if they display any developmental delays or disabilities.

The Elementary and Secondary Education Act (ESEA) was originally signed into law by former president Lyndon B. Johnson in 1965. It declared granting "full educational opportunity" a national priority. The law, reauthorized as NCLB in 2002, is being reconsidered once again. In January 2015, Secretary of Education Arne Duncan opened the door and invited Congress through it to create a law that would, among other goals, "foster innovation and advance equity."[15]

The time is ripe for such a vision. Now meditate on a remarkable story that lends a second-sighted, almost uncanny spin, to this juncture at which we stand. President Johnson's daughter Luci struggled for many years in school and was finally, at the age of sixteen, discovered to have poor eye coordination. In the account of her story, Luci shares that she was on the verge of dropping out of school when, as a last resort, the White House physician suggested she be seen by a local optometrist. She went through vision therapy, successfully completed high school, and later went on to graduate from college.[16]

The new Affordable Care Act is helping to pave the way. It's progressive in that the plan recognizes the need to go beyond the limited vision screening. This is the new standard under this coverage. It should serve as a model for all insurance carriers.[17]

While this is a huge step, there is more work to be done. We can no longer afford to have tunnel vision as a society. Community resources, ranging from schools to practitioners to families, must cooperate and harness the support, resources, and commitment needed to reach the *most vulnerable* of our children who don't have family support to get them the care they need.

"Leaders in business, education, government, health, and the nonprofit sector must come together to make vision care, including access to affordable prescription eyeglasses for all children, a priority in society. By doing so, a more literate society and a strong economic future may be ensured," Dr. Zaba writes in the online journal *Ophthalmology Times*.[18]

"The appropriate investment will require new partnerships to develop programs that provide health, social and educational programs that stress the importance of compliance," states Dr. Mozlin. "Appropriate infrastructures and systems will be required to ensure coordination and continuation of services. Innovations and strategies, such as school-based programs, must make these services available to the children, rather than waiting for parents to seek care for their children. A partnership of optometry, public health, and education might well have an impact on the high school drop-out rate by identifying students with vision problems, and providing them with the services they require."[19]

Partnership is a beautiful thing.

The National Commission on Vision and Health produced a report in cooperation with the Cambridge-based research firm Abt Associates, titled *Building a Comprehensive Child Vision System*. This work encompasses all of the elements needed to realize the vision that has been discussed throughout this book. Beginning with the rationale and moving through recommendations, guidelines, research, and an outlined plan of action, this report delineates in detail how to achieve the goal of reaching every child.[20]

A similar vision is described by Dr. Joel Zaba in his "Call to Action," articulately portrayed in a 2013 report by Barbara Obena for the AmeriCorps Child Vision Project. Specifically, he outlines a multilevel approach that includes action on a systemic level, an educator level, and a school-based level.

Both of these impressive resources are cited in the back of this book and provide the "how to" steps involved in working toward change. They are available online and can be reviewed and discussed at PTA and school board meetings and with leaders in education, health care, government, and business.[21]

Dr. Antonia Orfield has expressed her hope for such an aspiration. "If vision is a learned motor skill that is not being taught, and children are failing academic subjects, as well as becoming delinquent, illiterate, and learning disabled because they didn't acquire these basic skills first, then let us make sure that they do. If we know that low-powered, but necessary, reading glasses will not be obtained unless they are provided in the schools, then they need to be provided in the schools."[22]

Indeed, Dr. Orfield's passion, and that of many others who understand the importance of all that we have explored throughout this book, can be summed up in her words here: "I have a dream, a vision, really, about how every school should have the facilities for the vision development of children who come to school without their learning systems in place."[23]

After journeying through these pages, you may now envision the same dream. Until this dream becomes a reality, you have the knowledge to light the way and help the children in your life today.

A SPECIAL NOTE TO PARENTS AND TEACHERS

What do you do with all this newfound knowledge about the role that vision plays in learning and development? This likely will have had some measure of impact on your parenting and teaching philosophy.

Your creativity and good sense, along with a healthy dose of resourcefulness, can go very far in helping foster balance at home and in the classroom. You can help fortify children with little bites of sensory sustenance that will shore them up. Everyone will benefit from this.

Listed in the References section of this book are expert sources that will equip you with an abundance of ideas that will help you do this. In a general sense, what follow below are some guiding principles as you set off on this path.

Whenever you can, weave in time for stretching and movement. Take breaks often. Make it a game. Make it an intentional practice. Bring the kids on board with you as you finesse these sense-able measures into your day. It's likely they will soon become invested as they begin to feel the merits of awakening to their own senses.

Bring nature into your life. Plants and animals engage many senses and teach important values such as caring, responsibility, empathy, and respect. Display pictures of nature scenes. Play music with nature sounds. Bring activities outdoors as often as possible.

Encourage learning and discovery in 3-D (hands on and senses engaged) as opposed to 2-D (computers and screens).

And the children who always seem to stare out the window, get easily distracted from the task at hand, or ask to leave the classroom? Bear in mind that they may be creating an opportunity for themselves to relieve the stress they are under. They need an escape hatch in order to get by. Rather than viewing it as an annoyance and disruption, use it as both a clue and a cue.

If a child is classified, has accommodations, or is on medication for attention or behavior issues, have the child examined by a behavioral optometrist. If you're at the beginning stages of questioning what might be going on, simply have concerns, or are just not sure what to make of things, utilize the "Quality of Life Checklist" in Appendix A to see if the results indicate the need for further evaluation.

EPILOGUE

I have a very deep, personal appreciation for all specialty branches of the eye care profession. In addition to my experiences learning about vision-related learning problems as an adult, I've had an awareness of the different kinds of eye doctors from a very young age. When I was growing up, eye health terminology was household language.

My brother, Bruce Evan, who was four years younger than me, developed a rare form of pediatric eye cancer at the age of two. He lost his left eye to this. Fortunately, ophthalmologists were able to save his right eye, and therefore his vision, thanks to a progressive procedure.

Because he had one eye, he did not have binocular vision. He led a pretty normal life in spite of this, though he didn't participate much in sports since he did not have depth perception. Still, he was able to drive a car and went on to become an accomplished musician and, later on, a successful acupuncturist.

He used to say that he saw the world differently than most. He meant this literally since monocular vision will do that to a person. But he also meant that his experience, and the challenges that came with it, gave him a certain perspective that brought with it a heightened awareness of how fragile life is and an appreciation for what really matters.

He went on to survive a second bout with cancer in his twenties, brought on by the same gene mutation that caused the retinoblastoma when he was a toddler. Tragically, he succumbed to a third battle in 2007. He and I were not only siblings; we were extraordinarily close friends. His attitude continues to inspire me every day. Figuratively seeing the world through his eyes has helped shape my own views, which is perhaps why I cut to the chase and the heart of what matters most in just about any given situation.

I have little tolerance for trivialities that get in the way of permitting us all to be our best selves and live our best lives. Yet the reality is at times we're all affected by negative forces and compromised in some way. I think back on, with heartfelt difficulty, errors I made as an educator and faulty instances that occurred because of my own struggles with extensive systemic challenges that impeded my ability to be my best.

When we are able to learn from our experiences and obtain hindsight, though, we acquire wisdom that helps us move forward with a healthier, more sensitive consciousness and attentiveness. (If only there was vision therapy for lack of foresight that forces us to have to resort to hindsight!)

The pressure that many students and teachers are under to perform, each in their own realm, is crushing to the human spirit. It is a stumbling block and is at the root of many of society's most taxing concerns. We must look back with sobriety at the seeds we have sown and realize what we have grown. Then, with optimism and hope, we must look forward and commit to cultivating a new landscape.

We, as in *humanity*, need to put self-interests and rivalries aside and realize that we all need to help each other, starting foremost with our children. It's too depleting to slog through the swirl of counterproductivity and counterintuitiveness that limit our longing to flourish. We've heard government leaders declare in times of crisis that there shouldn't be any party lines, that everyone needs to work together so that we may save lives.

Really, though, it should always be about saving lives. It shouldn't have to come to a crisis. Imagine what we could accomplish if everyone came together for the greater good—always. How many lives affected by innumerable hidden crises that have become mundanely normative—though no less significant—would be saved?

The road ahead must acknowledge our arrival at a defining moment, indeed a crossroads, in our educational culture. We can no longer afford to look away from the injurious results of the unsustainable demands and expectations on our children. Ignoring their humanity and their limits will only come full circle and dramatically test our own. It already has.

My main goal for this book is to help children get the help they need by educating individuals and fostering much-needed awareness about this subject. Beyond this, my prevailing goal is to move toward creating systemic change. This change has to occur in two systems—education and health care. Vision lives in both domains, and this is a reality that deserves its due respect.

To move mountains, it will take all of us—parents, educators, doctors, lawyers, politicians, policy makers—our human village. Talk about this with everyone you know. Then gather specialties and skill sets, talents and fortes, and help kick our collective *visual figure ground* skills into high gear. We need to cut right through the irrelevant surrounding clutter and grab hold of what is needed. Now.

That is what this book is about.

AFTERWORD

See, I Am Smart by Wendy B. Rosen (2005)

I know that I'm smart.
There's so much that I know.
I can do lots of things
As I play, learn, and grow.
But sometimes I struggle.
It just all seems so tough.
I am doing my best,
But it's just not enough.
My teachers, my parents
Just don't seem to know
Why school is so hard,
Why my grades are so low.
Then one day we learned
That my eyes didn't see
The way they're supposed to.
Who knew? Not even me!
I thought everyone saw
Letters dancing and clumping,
The words in 3-D,
The sentences jumping.
As I read through a page,
I would soon lose my way.
I would have to start over.
This took me all day!

I never quite knew
Why it took me so long
To do all my work,
Then get so much wrong.
But now we have answers.
I now know it's not me.
It's just that my eyes
Confuse that which I see.
Thankfully, though,
We have learned there's a way
To help teach my eyes
To see better each day.
It will take some hard work
And some time to achieve,
But I know it'll be worth it.
This much I believe.
My eyes and my brain
Now work out every day.
Vision therapy isn't easy,
But I know it's the way.
It'll help train my eyes
To perceive the world right
So that I'll understand
All that is in my sight.
With my vision corrected,
I know now I will soar.
I will reach my potential.
I will struggle no more.
I am smart; don't you see?
There's so much I can do.
I will be a success,
And I'm proud of me, too!

ACKNOWLEDGMENTS

This has been by far the hardest part of the book to write, as I don't know how to adequately put into words my thanks and gratitude to so many people who have been a part of this extraordinary journey with me. Without you, my work and this book would not have been possible. I'll begin where it all began.

My deepest, heartfelt appreciation goes to Dr. Linda Tamm for setting us on the right path and launching this life-changing journey for all of us. My gratitude to you is infinite; my respect for you runs deep.

Enormous thanks go to Dr. William Moskowitz, for your gentle manner and profound expertise and wisdom, and to Nan Miller for your guidance and mentorship. Your combined inspiration has continued to propel me forward with this important work to this day.

To Karen Kanter and Steve Heisler, I owe immense thanks for initially reaching out and then reaching out some more on my behalf, enabling me to become an author. I will be forever grateful to you both for this gift.

For your deeply valued involvement and contribution, my warmest thanks and appreciation go to Brian Selznick and Noel Silverman.

To Tom Koerner, Carlie Wall, and Lara Graham at Rowman & Littlefield, I feel so fortunate to have you as my editors. Your patience, guidance, reliance, and confidence in my writing buoyed me throughout this exhilarating adventure and for this I am deeply grateful.

Over the many years I have been doing this work, I've had the privilege of building connections with remarkable individuals who have given me support, encouragement, and opportunities to learn. To Bob Williams, Dr. Maureen Powers, Dr. S. Moshe Roth, Toni Bristol, Janet Hughes, Laurie Anderson, and Debbie Miller, I extend my sincere appreciation.

There are so many people who have played key roles at various junctures along the path as this book unfolded. I've had the great honor of consulting with many top professionals across disciplines who have so generously given of their time and expertise. I have felt embraced and anchored by their assurance and enthusiasm for my efforts. I extend my deepest respect, admiration, and gratitude to Dr. Leonard Press, Dr. Nancy Torgerson, Dr. Thomas Lenart, Dr. Paul Harris, Dr. Lynn Hellerstein, Dr. Sue Cotter, Dr. Rochelle Mozlin, Dr. Kirti Patel, Dr. Joel Zaba, Dr. Susan Barry, Dr. Stacy Lyons, Dr. Brenda Montecalvo, Dr. Josh Watt, Robert Nurisio, Dr. Marcy Guddemi, Dr. William Padula, Dr. Jonathon Jenness, Jackie Haines, Dr. Carl Hillier, Dr. Claude Valenti, Katie Johnson, Sara Bennett, Dr. Carla Hannaford, Dr. William Crain, Carol Kranowitz, Joye Newman, Jayne Wesler, Patricia Lemer, Dr. Richard Rothstein, Dr. Deborah Walker, and Rae Pica.

Huge thanks go out to the wonderful staff at Eyecare Professionals, Traci-Lin and the wonderful staff at Family Eyecare Associates, Kelin Kushin, Theresa Krejci, and Michael Beberman for providing logistic support.

I am very grateful to Dr. Maurice Elias, Dr. Jeffrey Kress, Jordan Siegel, Dr. Chonita Spencer, Anita Hall-Kane, Robin Benoit, Valerie Pessirilo, and Roz Beberman for your part that helped shape the whole.

Dr. Amy Kavanaugh, Dr. Wayne Rebarber, Rachelle Rebarber, Stacey Narula, Shoshanna Katzman, Howard and Beth Cannon, and Dr. Marc DeVito—you will always have my warmest, heartfelt gratitude.

Dr. Barry Tannen, I am so grateful for your expertise and top-notch care that you provide to my family. Beyond this, your support and encouragement throughout this process, from its infancy, has been my mainstay and I owe you a wealth of thanks.

To the parents and children who have shared your stories with me, I congratulate you for the victories you have achieved and extend my warmest thanks to you for trusting me with your words. You have played an important role in helping others learn about this.

Thank you to my mother-in-law and father-in-law, Janice and Gerald Rosen, for your quiet thoughtfulness, enthusiasm for my writing, and support always.

Thank you to my mom, Ella, for your positive energy and incredible strength that provide a beacon in my life, for always believing in me, and for being my biggest cheerleader.

Sara and Jonah, thank you for being two of the most wonderful children a parent could hope for. You fill me with pride for so many reasons and continue to amaze me as you grow. I am an incredibly lucky mom.

Mitchel, thank you for your love, your unending patience and unwavering support that manifested in so many ways, for believing in me, and my work, and for keeping our household running while I was absorbed in birthing this book.

APPENDIX A

Symptoms Checklist

Quality of Life Checklist

College of
Optometrists in
Vision Development
Prevention · Enhancement · Rehabilitation

Patient Name: _____

Form Completed by: _____

Date: _____

Check the column which best represents the occurrence of each symptom	Never 0	Seldom 1	Occasionally 2	Frequently 3	Always 4
Blurred close vision					
Double vision					
Headaches with near work					
Words run together reading					
Burning, itchy, watery eyes					
Falls asleep reading					
Sees worse at the end of day					
Skips/repeats lines reading					
Dizzy/nauseated by near work					
Head tilt/one eye closed to read					
Difficulty copying from chalkboard					
Avoids near work/reading					
Omits small words when reading					
Writes uphill/downhill					
Misaligns digits/columns of numbers					
Poor reading comprehension					
Poor/inconsistent in sports					
Holds reading too close					
Trouble keeping attention on reading					
Difficulty completing work on time					
Says "I can't" before trying					
Avoids sports/games					
Poor hand/eye coordination					
Poor handwriting					
Does not judge distance accurately					
Clumsy, knocks things over					
Poor time use/management					
Does not make change well					
Loses things/belongings					
Car or motion sickness					
Forgetfulness/poor memory					
Total for each column:					
Grand Total:					

<15 = Routine eye exam recommended   **16-24** = Comprehensive exam with developmental OD recommended   **>25** = Developmental vision problem likely, comprehensive exam with developmental OD strongly recommended

215 W. Garfield Rd, Suite 200 Aurora, OH 44202 | 330-995-0718 | www.covd.org

Quality-of-Life Checklist

APPENDIX B

Sharing Stories

Until one has personally witnessed how life changing vision therapy can be for a struggling child, when no other strategies have helped that child, it is hard to get a real sense of the relief, empowerment, and confidence that children and their families feel. This section is composed entirely of personal stories as told by children who went through it and by parents who supported them.

There are perhaps no other more inspiring words on the subject than those you are about to read.

My son Michael has completed vision therapy. This school year he has made several improvements. Michael has become a more confident reader. He does not skip lines. He reads more fluently and his spelling has improved. Michael's handwriting has also improved—it is more legible. Reversals are not as frequent. Michael also feels more confident in class, which makes him eager to participate. His comprehension grade has improved. He has been able to read both to me and on his own with more understanding of the story. He will read a book to me, on his level, and ask me comprehension questions!

—Michael's dad

Elise was not reading when we started vision therapy. She couldn't read anything beyond a three-letter word. She can now read words over five letters and has jumped several reading levels. She has become a lot more confident too. Elise also wants to read and wants to learn—something she didn't want to do before.

—Elise's dad

I can see easier. I can read more and I am better at baseball. I can see the board at school easier, and I can read without my eyes hurting. It helped me with everything overall.

—Jeffrey

The changes are remarkable. Jeffrey has improved at least two reading levels. His grades have improved as well as his willingness to read. Instead of complaining of a stomachache and going to the school nurse to avoid reading, he volunteers to read out loud. Jeffrey's confidence has greatly increased. The changes happened so quickly. He had used his finger to read and within the first month we noticed it stopped. It is such a joy to watch him read and discuss a book with us. This is something we were beginning to think would never happen.

In addition to reading, his math grades have improved too. Just recently he was asked to participate in the sixth-grade math contest. We are still waiting for the results but are still excited that he was asked. This has been a life-changing experience for him, and it has made his life so much better.

—Jeffrey's dad

I noticed that I improved at many things that were hard in vision therapy. I also noticed that I can tell when I'm switching eyes and when I'm using them together. My batting improved because vision therapy is helping me see with two eyes. It changed my life. Vision therapy makes you feel more confident.

—Becky

Ethan has become more confident in his reading abilities. He does not struggle as much at school. He is now able to hit a baseball as well. Ethan uses both eyes when he reads now rather than just one. It was a huge relief to finally have answers for why he was struggling so much with school.

—Ethan's dad

Daniel is now able to read with much less fatigue. Before he started vision therapy to address his convergence insufficiency, he would tire after just a page of reading (even if he was interested in it) and would ask me to read it to him. Now, Daniel will read a chapter without complaint and if he really likes a book, will read without being asked— unheard of before VT.

In addition, before VT, Daniel would not attempt to do schoolwork that had a lot of problems or reading material on the page—it was too overwhelming. Now, he doesn't refuse and he does not seem to have any anxiety about it. His vision is no longer "double," and he can read without fatiguing early on.

—Daniel's dad

Max is so much better coordinated! He is not falling as much or bumping into walls. He is finally peeing into the toilet because he has depth perception now! And he is happy to do his fun vision exercises now. He is even starting to have more interest in fine motor things—letters, numbers, and learning in general. I am very critical of therapists because we have been through so many with my older child, and Max is only three and a half, but the vision therapist made everything fun.

—Max's mom

By the time my daughter Tricia turned five, it was clear to me that reading was going to be a struggle for her. She was an early talker and always verbally advanced. She is also quite emotionally intelligent. I had watched her older siblings and twin brother learn to read easily, as if one day a switch just flipped. When she started kindergarten at an excellent Montessori school, Tricia was still having trouble writing her name and identifying all sound symbol relationships.

Despite months of review and practice, she just didn't seem to make much progress. In first grade, she really began to fall behind. She was lucky to be born with a healthy dose of self-confidence, and this got her through many months of frustration. By the spring, as her peers began to read simple chapter books, she was still making her way through phonics readers and was beginning to hate school.

She started to work with a reading specialist, and although she made some good progress, reading still was too hard. Around this time, she also began complaining of headaches and was growing frequently restless, often asking for bathroom breaks or trips to the water fountain. Her teachers were also growing increasingly frustrated. They felt Tricia was too smart to have learning issues and that she was too headstrong, too lazy, or too focused on her creative passions to really care about school. As a clinical psychologist who has a private testing practice and knows how complex learning profiles can be, I knew better. But I couldn't figure out what was going on.

One day towards the end of the school year, I was meeting with a family whose daughter I had recommended to a vision therapist. I invited Wendy into the meeting, as I knew this was her area of expertise and thought she could be a great resource for any questions they might have about the process. As I listened to her talk, it suddenly dawned on me that Tricia was struggling with many of the things she was talking about and that perhaps she too could benefit from vision therapy.

The next week I brought Tricia in for an evaluation, and sure enough, she had significant visual challenges and was recommended for a thirty-six-session course of treatment. Tricia has been in treatment since September of this school year, and she is about to finish next month. If you ask her about it, she would say that vision therapy "literally changed my life." She has made so much progress this year and is reading at or close to her second-grade level. She feels like a "good student" and says this is the best year she has ever had in school. I am so grateful for this therapeutic intervention and know that we have set her up for success. We are looking forward to a great third-grade year!

—Tricia's mom

Harrison was seeing double up to a distance of forty-four inches, and with vision therapy, this had reduced down to three inches. At the beginning of his school year, his handwriting was very poor and he even had a very difficult time recognizing sight words. He had to tap out all the words. Harrison is now reading without tapping out the words and even with emotion. His confidence has also improved and his self-esteem has built up too, as he is so happy and proud that he can read now.

—Harrison's parents

I always loved music. I had taken piano lessons starting at age three, learned flute in fifth grade, and played xylophone in my middle-school band. But as much music as I played, I always had a hard time quickly reading the notes, making it harder for me to learn the music and having it take longer too. I was also seeing objects in double vision, which I believed was normal.

One day during an OT (occupational therapy) exam, the therapist noticed that there was something off with my eyes. She recommended vision therapy to us to fix the problem. We went to the eye doctor, and it was found that I had a convergence issue.

After a year of vision therapy, it was determined that my convergence issue was fixed. Now I don't see double vision anymore, and I can read sheet music so much easier. Vision therapy has opened so many more doors for me; I don't know where I'd be now without it.

—Emily

Matthew continues to improve his skills with each semester. He is completing the fourth grade, and his fluency is on grade level! We are confident his comprehension and writing skills will follow that trend.

—Matthew's mom

When Jenny was classified as having a nonspecific learning disability in seventh grade, it was very upsetting to us all. Getting classified in seventh grade is an awful thing. Getting switched to a different learning track and becoming a special needs student impacts self-esteem.

I had first questioned teachers in third grade, when she received a "below proficient" score on the New Jersey ASK standardized test. The low score did not match the 96 percent average she had on her report card. Over the course of five years, I kept questioning teachers about inconsistencies I saw with Jenny. She would get the last few answers on tests wrong. Little did we know that her vision became blurred after just a few pages because her eyes were so tired.

She would fall asleep each and every time she sat down to read. Family members labeled her lazy. I brought her to counseling since she often felt frustrated doing her homework, which took forever to complete every night. Children, of course, do not realize this is abnormal. They just deal with it, and they become frustrated.

Four months of vision therapy gave her the tools she needed to succeed. She was able to read texts and focus better on the computer. She also understood why she had such great difficulties.

She now has a 94 percent average again and was inducted into the Junior National Honor Society. Jenny is on a much better path now because of vision therapy.

—Jenny's mom

I used to be unable to catch a Frisbee, hit a softball and baseball, and even simply throw a ball up and then successfully catch it. My hand-eye coordination was never great. With strabismus added to that, most sports were difficult to enjoy. Focusing on nearby objects was never easy as well. By the time I finished VT, I was able to play many sports just as well as my peers, and seeing double only occurred with carbon-copy pages and kaleidoscopes. My focus is significantly better, and it is much easier to coordinate everything.

—Joey

I went through vision therapy when I was in elementary school. I learned how to process information so I could understand what I was being taught. I used what I learned in vision therapy and am now entering my senior year at Marist College.

—Andrew

Since beginning vision therapy, I've noticed now I don't tire as fast while I am reading. My headaches are very rare. I can read for longer periods of time without getting vertigo or headaches. My vertigo is very seldom. I do not reread sentences numerous times.

—Zoe, adult TBI patient

NOTES

PREFACE

1. Retrieved April 24, 2014, from http://www.visionandlearning.org.

1. THE DIFFERENCE BETWEEN VISION AND EYESIGHT

1. Moskowitz, D. W. (2004). Interviewer: W. Rosen.

2. Retrieved September 1, 2015, from http://museumofvision.org/dynamic/files/uploaded_files_filename_157.pdf.

3. Hannaford, C. (2005). *Smart Moves: Why Learning Is Not All In Your Head*. Salt Lake City, Utah: Great River Books.

4. Retrieved May 7, 2014, from https://www.nei.nih.gov/sites/default/files/nei-pdfs/SeeAllYouCanSeeCalendar.pdf. Retrieved September 30, 2015, from http://www.smithsonianmag.com/science-nature/why-do-we-blink-so-frequently-172334883/?no-ist.

5. Weil, A. (1999). *Breathing: The Master Key to Self Healing*. Boulder, Colorado: Sounds True, Inc.

6. Retrieved October 30, 2015, from http://www.aoa.org/patients-and-public/good-vision-throughout-life/childrens-vision/infant-vision-birth-to-24-months-of-age?sso=y.

7. Retrieved March 24, 2014, from http://www.visionandlearning.org/visionexam08.html.

8. Retrieved May 7, 2014, from https://www.nei.nih.gov/sites/default/files/nei-pdfs/SeeAllYouCanSeeCalendar.pdf; September 1, 2015, from http://www.

aoa.org/patients-and-public/caring-for-your-vision/comprehensive-eye-and-vision-examination?sso=y; March 30, 2014, from http://www.visionandlearning.org/visionexam08.html; April 24, 2014, from http://www.visionandlearning.org; March 30, 2015, from http://www.childrensvision.com/reading.htm.

9. Retrieved August 25, 2015, from http://www.sciencedaily.com/releases/2008/07/080703145849.htm.

10. Orfield, A. (2007). *Eyes for Learning: Preventing and Curing Vision-Related Learning Problems*. Lanham, Maryland: Rowman & Littlefield.

11. Hellerstein, L. (2010). *See It. Say It. Do It!* Centennial, Colorado: Hi-Clear Publishing.

2. WHAT ARE VISION-RELATED LEARNING PROBLEMS?

1. Retrieved August 25, 2015, from http://visionhelp.org/perceptually-impaired-now-what.

2. Retrieved May 6, 2015, from http://ophthalmologytimes.modernmedicine.com/ophthalmologytimes/content/many-children-today-lack-good-vision-care?page=full.

3. Retrieved August 25, 2015, from http://www.covd.org/?page=August_VL.

4. Retrieved August 25, 2015, from http://www.visionandlearning.org/visionandlearning08.html.

5. Retrieved August 25, 2015, from http://www.covd.org/?page=August_VL.

6. *Current Ophthalmology, 43*(5), March–April 1999, 445–457.

7. Retrieved June 2, 2015, from http://devdelay.org/newsletter/vol11-num4-06-summer.pdf.

8. Retrieved December 3, 2014, from http://www.ncld.org.

9. Wilmhurst, L., and Brue, L. (2005). *A Parent's Guide to Special Education: Insider Advice on How to Navigate the System and Help Your Child Succeed*. New York: AMACOM.

10. Retrieved March 26, 2015, from http://visionhelp.org/osu-researchers-find-conclusive-link-between-vision-problems-and-children-with-ieps.

11. *The Vision Council Report: Making the Grade*, 2009, 1–24.

12. Garzia, R. (2008). *Care of the Patient with Learning Related Vision Problems Optometric Clinical Practice Guideline*. St. Louis, Missouri: American Optometric Association; p. 38.

13. Brenne Henke, M., and Greenburg, R. M. (1985). Learning Related Visual Problems. In E. C. o. H. a. G. Children (Ed.), (pp. 2). https://

archive.org/stream/ERIC_ED309582#page/n1/mode/2up. Garzia, *Care of the Patient*, 38. Retrieved March 30, 2014, from http://www.visionandlearning.org/visionexam08.html. Retrieved August 26, 2015, from http://www.covd.org/?page=symptoms. Retrieved March 30, 2015, from http://www.childrensvision.com/reading.htm. Torgerson, N. (2002). How Perceptual Skills May Affect Learning. *Consulting With Schools: Behavioral Aspects of Vision Care, 42*(3), 72.

14. Retrieved October 30, 2015, from http://www.aoa.org/patients-and-public/good-vision-throughout-life/childrens-vision/infant-vision-birth-to-24-months-of-age?sso=y.

15. Orfield, A. (2007). *Eyes for Learning: Preventing and Curing Vision-Related Learning Problems*. Lanham, Maryland: Rowman & Littlefield; p. 243.

16. Hannaford, C. (2005). *Smart Moves: Why Learning Is Not All in Your Head*. Salt Lake City, Utah: Great River Books; pp. 35–37.

17. Appelbaum, S. A., and Hoopes, A. M. (2009). *Eye Power*. Dr. Stanley A. Appelbaum and Ann M. Hoopes; p. 18.

18. Retrieved April 28, 2015, from http://www.npr.org/2014/03/08/287255411/what-the-u-s-can-learn-from-finland-where-school-starts-at-age-7.

19. Retrieved April 28, 2015, from http://news.stanford.edu/news/2012/january/finnish-schools-reform-012012.html; http://www.smithsonianmag.com/innovation/why-are-finlands-schools-successful-49859555/?no-ist; and http://www.edweek.org/tm/articles/2014/06/24/ctq_faridi_finland.html.

20. Pica, R. (2015). *What if Everybody Understood Child Development? Straight Talk About Bettering Education and Children's Lives*. Thousand Oaks, California: Corwin Press; pp. 6–7.

21. Retrieved May 8, 2015, from http://www.allianceforchildhood.org/sites/allianceforchildhood.org/files/file/Crisis_%20flier.pdf.

22. Jackson, M. (2005, July 17). Don't Let the TV Be the Baby Sitter. *Sunday Boston Globe*.

23. http://www.ncbi.nlm.nih.gov/pmc/articles/PMC155411/.

24. Retrieved August 26, 2015, from http://www.concussionproject.com/.

25. Retrieved May 6, 2015, from http://newsnetwork.mayoclinic.org/discussion/mayo-clinic-researchers-validate-rapid-sideline-concussion-test-for-youth-athletes. Retrieved May 6, 2015, from http://us1.campaign-archive2.com/?u=5677da6a1cc2a453899683120&id=398932a39f&e=ab7f97c848.

3. "WHY HAVEN'T I HEARD ABOUT THIS BEFORE?"

1. Retrieved September 9, 2015, from http://psycnet.apa.org/psycinfo/1994-38578-001.

2. Retrieved September 9, 2015, from http://psycnet.apa.org/psycinfo/ 1994-38578-001.

3. Retrieved November 4, 2014, from http://www.optometrists.org/ therapists_teachers/PTA_reading_vision_learn.html.

4. Seiderman, A. S. (1989). *20/20 Is Not Enough: The New World of Vision*. New York: Alfred A. Knopf; p. 68.

5. Seiderman, *20/20 Is Not Enough*, 9.

6. Hannaford, C. (2005). *Smart Moves: Why Learning Is Not All In Your Head*. Salt Lake City, Utah: Great River Books; p. 52.

4. "BUT I WAS TOLD THIS IS A BUNCH OF HOOEY!"

1. Retrieved May 6, 2015, from http://www.children-special-needs.org/ parenting/pediatric_opthalmologist.html.

2. Retrieved November 19, 2014, from http://www.nytimes.com/2010/03/ 14/magazine/14vision-t.html?pagewanted=all&_r=0.

3. Retrieved November 20, 2014, from http://www.fvdcpc.com/pdf/ important-new-research.pdf.

4. Retrieved May 15, 2015, from https://www.nei.nih.gov/news/ pressreleases/101308.

5. Retrieved October 27, 2014, from http://www.fvdcpc.com/pdf/the-effectiveness-of-vision-therapy.pdf.

6. Retrieved October 27, 2014, from http://www.fvdcpc.com/pdf/the-effectiveness-of-vision-therapy.pdf.

7. Katzman, S. (2003). *Qigong for Staying Young*. New York: Penguin Group.

8. Retrieved August 27, 2015, from http://www.allaboutvision.com/cvs/ children-computer-vision-syndrome.htm.

9. Retrieved August 27, 2015, from https://www.acbo.org.au/for-patients/ your-questions-answered/what-is-vision-therapy.

10. Retrieved August 27, 2015, from http://www.pressvision.com/family_ eyecare_associates_research.php.

11. Retrieved February 8, 2015, from http://www.children-special-needs. org/parenting/pediatric_opthalmologist.html.

12. Retrieved November 20, 2014, from http://www.aapos.org/terms/ conditions/108.

13. Retrieved May 11, 2015, from http://www.hopkinsmedicine.org/wilmer/ news/sightline/Sightline_Special_Edition_Annual_Report_2014.pdf.

14. Retrieved December 2, 2014, from http://lynnhellerstein.com/wp-content/uploads/2013/03/ICDL-guidelines-Chapter-11-written-by-OMD.pdf.

15. Retrieved December 5, 2014, from http://ht.ly/p1QgZ.

5. SENSORY OVERLOAD

1. Retrieved May 6, 2015, from http://ophthalmologytimes.modernmedicine.com/ophthalmologytimes/content/many-children-today-lack-good-vision-care?page=full.

2. Retrieved January 11, 2015, from http://www.ascd.org/publications/books/104013/chapters/Movement-and-Learning.aspx.

3. Retrieved January 12, 2015, from http://www.braingym.org/history.

4. Hannaford, C. (2005). *Smart Moves: Why Learning Is Not All In Your Head*. Salt Lake City, Utah: Great River Books; p. 20.

5. Bennett, S., and Kalish, N. (2006). *The Case Against Homework*. New York: Crown Publishers; pp. 23–27.

6. Retrieved June 3, 2015, from http://www.alfiekohn.org/teaching/dwh.htm.

7. Retrieved May 11, 2015, from http://www.ascd.org/publications/educational-leadership/mar07/vol64/num06/The-Case-For-and-Against-Homework.aspx. Retrieved May 11, 2015, from http://www.challengesuccess.org/Portals/0/Docs/ChallengeSuccess-DoYouKnow-Elementary.pdf.

8. Retrieved May 11, 2015, from http://www.challengesuccess.org.

9. Bennett and Kalish, *The Case Against Homework*, 95–97.

10. Retrieved February 9, 2015, from http://www.sciencedaily.com/releases/2015/02/150202123716.htm.

11. Retrieved February 10, 2015, from https://www.psychologytoday.com/blog/child-sleep-zzzs/201406/new-evidence-sleep-facilitates-learning-and-memory.

12. Retrieved February 12, 2015, from https://teensneedsleep.files.wordpress.com/2011/03/carskadon-when-worlds-collide.pdf.

13. Retrieved August 28, 2015, from http://www.oed.com/view/Entry/227459?redirectedFrom=wellness#eid.

14. Retrieved May 18, 2015, from http://eric.ed.gov/?id=ED119389.

15. Orfield, A. (2007). *Eyes for Learning: Preventing and Curing Vision-Related Learning Problems*. Lanham, Maryland: Rowman & Littlefield; pp. 118–126.

16. Orfield, *Eyes for Learning*, 97–98.

17. Retrieved February 15, 2015, from http://cdn2.hubspot.net/hub/91892/file-15972053-pdf/docs/sarah_cobb_harmon_revisited.pdf.

18. Retrieved February 15, 2015, from http://cdn2.hubspot.net/hub/91892/file-15972053-pdf/docs/sarah_cobb_harmon_revisited.pdf.

19. Retrieved May 18, 2015, from http://oepf.org/sites/default/files/Easier%20More%20Productive%20Study%20and%20Desk%20Work.pdf.

20. Hannaford, *Smart Moves*, 116–117.

21. Hannaford, *Smart Moves*, 119.

22. Hannaford, *Smart Moves*, 40–41.

23. Hannaford, *Smart Moves*, 113–114.

24. Hannaford, *Smart Moves*, 119.

6. CHANGING LIVES

1. Catalyst Vision and Learning Education Kit. (2002). Encinatas, California: Catalyst Solutions, L.L.C.

2. Retrieved February 25, 2015, from http://visionhelp.org/visionacademic-problems-and-the-emotional-fallout. Retrieved March 23, 2015, from http://www.wrightslaw.com/info/jj.delinq.read.probs.htm.

3. Wheeler, T. A., and McQuarrie, C. W. (1992). Vision, Juvenile Delinquency and Learning Disabilities. *Behavioral Aspects of Vision Care, 41*(3), 1–9.

4. Shapiro, S. Vision and Juvenile Delinquency. https://www.ncjrs.gov/App/Publications/abstract.aspx?ID=54020.

5. Dzik, D. (2000). Behavioral Optometric Vision: A Practical and Comprehensive Plan for Juvenile Delinquency Control. *Behavioral Aspects of Vision Care, 41*(3), 30–35.

6. Dzik, Behavioral Optometric Vision, 30–35.

7. Wheeler and McQuarrie, Vision, Juvenile Delinquency and Learning Disabilities, 1–9. Lecoq, T. (2000). Vision and Juvenile Delinquency: A Compilation of Results of Optometric Intervention Programs Conducted in Juvenile Delinquents' Detention Facilities. *Behavioral Aspects of Vision Care, 41*(3), 76–80. Harris, P. (2000). The Prevalence of Visual Conditions in a Population of Juvenile Delinquents. *Behavioral Aspects of Vision Care, 41*(3), 57–75.

8. Zaba, J. N. (2011). Children's Vision Care in the 21st Century & Its Impact on Education, Literacy, Social Issues, & the Workplace: A Call to Action. *Journal of Behavioral Optometry, 22*(2), 39–41.

9. Retrieved September 2, 2015, from http://www.wrightslaw.com/info/jj.delinq.read.probs.htm.

10. Retrieved September 2, 2015, from http://www.wrightslaw.com/info/jj.delinq.read.probs.htm.

11. Wheeler and McQuarrie, Vision, Juvenile Delinquency and Learning Disabilities, 1–9.

12. Retrieved May 12, 2015, from http://oepf.org/sites/default/files/Juvenile%20Delinquents%20Paul%20Harris.pdf.

13. Retrieved May 12, 2015, from http://www.pbs.org/wgbh/pages/frontline/shows/juvenile/bench/whatittakes.html.

14. Johnson, R. A., and Zaba, J. N. (2000). The Visual Screening of Adjudicated Adolescents. *Behavioral Aspects of Vision Care, 41*(3), 36–41.

15. Zaba, J. N. (2001). Social, Emotional, and Educational Consequences of Undetected Children's Vision Problems. *Journal of Behavioral Optometry, 12*(3), 66–69.

16. Zaba, Social, Emotional, and Educational Consequences, 66–69.

17. Wheeler and McQuarrie, Vision, Juvenile Delinquency and Learning Disabilities, 1–9. Johnson, R. (2000). "How To" Information and Success Stories. *Behavioral Aspects of Vision Care, 41*(3), 47–54.

18. Zaba, Social, Emotional, and Educational Consequences, 66–69.

19. Zaba, Children's Vision Care in the 21st Century, 39–41.

20. Severtson, R. (2000). Screening and Treatment Program for Vision and Learning Disabilities among Juvenile Delinquents. *Behavioral Aspects of Vision Care, 41*(3), 42–46.

21. From Wilder, T., Allgood, W., and Rothstein, R. (2008). *Narrowing the Achievement Gap for Low-Income Children: A 19-Year Life Cycle Approach.* New York: Teachers College, Columbia University.

22. Retrieved March 30, 2015, from http://www.optometrists.org/therapists_teachers/NAACP_Resolution_Vision_Therapy_High_Risk.html. Retrieved March 30, 2015, from http://www.add-adhd.org/at_risk_at-risk_students.html.

23. Retrieved April 21, 2015, from http://www.aoa.org/news/healthcare-reform/aoas-push-for-eye-care-for-children-continues-?sso=y.

24. Barry, S. R. (2009). *Fixing My Gaze.* New York: Basic Books.

25. Benoit, R. (2012). *Jillian's Story: How Vision Therapy Changed My Daughter's Life.* Dallas, Texas: The Small Press. Benoit, R. (2013). *Dear Jillian: Vision Therapy Changed My Life Too.* Dallas, Texas: The Small Press.

26. Retrieved May 10, 2015, from http://www.oepf.org/sites/default/files/journals/jbo-volume-12-issue-3/12-3%20Guest%20Editorial.pdf.

27. Retrieved May 10, 2015, from http://www.optometrists.org/therapists_teachers/Harvard_study_literacy.html.Retrieved May 10, 2015, from http://www.oepf.org/sites/default/files/journals/jbo-volume-12-issue-3/12-3%20Guest%20Editorial.pdf.

7. THEIR FUTURE, OUR FUTURE

1. Padula, W. V. (2012). *Neuro-Visual Processing Rehabilitation: An Interdisciplinary Approach*. Santa Ana, California: Optometric Extension Program Foundation; p. 100.

2. Gesell, A. (2014). *Vision: Its Development in Infant and Child*. New York: Asian Press; p. 51.

3. Retrieved April 22, 2015, from http://www.childstudycenter.yale.edu/centennial/exhibit/gesell.aspx.

4. Gesell, *Vision*, 20.

5. Retrieved April 23, 2015, from http://www.health.harvard.edu/press_releases/light-from-laptops-tvs-electronics-and-energy-efficient-lightbulbs-may-harm-health.

6. Retrieved April 24, 2015, from http://www.who.int/mediacentre/factsheets/fs311/en/.

7. Crain, W. (2003). *Reclaiming Childhood*. New York: Henry Holt and Company; p. 1.

8. Pappano, L. (February 8, 2015). Is Your First Grader College Ready? Education. *The New York Times*, pp. 12–15.

9. Crain, *Reclaiming Childhood*, 155.

10. Quoted in Crain, *Reclaiming Childhood*, 11–14.

11. Quoted in Crain, *Reclaiming Childhood*, 181.

12. Retrieved April 15, 2015, from http://neatoday.org/2013/04/25/a-nation-at-risk-turns-30-where-did-it-take-us-2/.

13. Retrieved April 15, 2015, from http://www.asha.org/Advocacy/federal/nclb/exec-summary/.

14. Retrieved April 15, 2015, from http://www.npr.org/blogs/ed/2015/04/13/398804901/senators-try-to-revise-no-child-left-behind-a-few-years-behind.

15. Retrieved April 15, 2015, from https://www.whitehouse.gov/the-press-office/fact-sheet-race-top.

16. Retrieved April 15, 2015, from http://www.boldapproach.org/report. Retrieved April 15, 2015, from http://www2.ed.gov/nclb/overview/intro/execsumm.html. Retrieved April 15, 2015, from http://www.npr.org/blogs/ed/2015/04/13/398804901/senators-try-to-revise-no-child-left-behind-a-few-years-behind.

17. Retrieved April 22, 2015, from http://www.childstudycenter.yale.edu/centennial/exhibit/gesell.aspx.

18. Gesell, *Vision*, 18–21, 23–29, 33, 45.

19. Gesell, *Vision*, 71–73.

20. Gesell, *Vision*, 74–77, 84–88.

21. Gesell, *Vision*, 431–433.

22. Gesell Institute of Child Development. (2013–2014). *Annual Report.* New Haven, Connecticut: Gesell Institute of Child Development; p. 7. Gesell Institute of Child Development. (2010). *Gesell's Guide for Parents and Teachers: Understanding the Relationship Between Families and Schools.* New Haven, Connecticut: Gesell Institute of Child Development.

23. Abeles, V. (2009). *Race to Nowhere.* Reel Link Films. Retrieved April 19, 2015, from http://www.racetonowhere.com/rtn-story.

8. A VISION FOR LEARNING

1. Retrieved April 22, 2015, from http://www.jcu.edu.au/wiledpack/modules/fsl/JCU_090460.html.

2. Retrieved April 22, 2015, from http://www.washingtonpost.com/blogs/answer-sheet/wp/2013/10/16/howard-gardner-multiple-intelligences-are-not-learning-styles/.

3. Retrieved April 22, 2015, from http://www.ascd.org/publications/books/100006/chapters/The-Theory-of-Multiple-Intelligences.aspx.

4. Gardner, H. (1993). *Multiple Intelligences: The Theory in Practice.* New York: Basic Books; pp. 84–85.

5. Retrieved September 4, 2015, from http://www.washingtonpost.com/blogs/answer-sheet/wp/2015/03/27/as-testing-opt-out-movement-grows-so-does-pushback-from-schools/.

6. Ilg, F. L., and Ames, L. B. (1978). *School Readiness: Behavior Tests Used at the Gesell Institute.* New York: Harper Collins; p. 241.

7. Zaba, J. N., Mozlin, R., and Reynolds, W. T. (2003). Insights on the Efficacy of Vision Examinations and Vision Screenings for Children First Entering School. *Journal of Behavioral Optometry, 14*(5), 123–126.

8. Retrieved May 13, 2015, from http://oepf.org/sites/default/files/journals/jbo-volume-14-issue-5/14-5%20ZabaReynolds.pdf.

9. Retrieved May 13, 2015, from http://www.healthypeople.gov/2020/topics-objectives/topic/vision/objectives. Retrieved May 13, 2015, from http://www.healthypeople.gov/2020/tools-resources/evidence-based-resource/visual-acuity-screening-children.

10. Zaba, J. N. (2011). Children's Vision Care in the 21st Century & Its Impact on Education, Literacy, Social Issues, & the Workplace: A Call to Action. *Journal of Behavioral Optometry, 22*(2), 39–41.

11. Zaba, Mozlin, and Reynolds, Insights on the Efficacy of Vision Examinations, 123–126.

12. Retrieved May 11, 2015, from http://www.ncbi.nlm.nih.gov/pubmed/21923871.

13. Mozlin, R. (2001). Poverty, Neurodevelopment and Vision: A Demonstration Project with an Adolescent Population. *Journal of Behavioral Optometry, 12*(3), 71–74.

14. Retrieved May 13, 2015, from http://ajot.aota.org/article.aspx?articleid=1881635.

15. Retrieved May 13, 2015, from http://www.ed.gov/esea.

16. Nugent, L. J. (2000). *I Was Nearly A Dropout* (Vol. #A103). Santa Ana, California: Optometric Extension Program Foundation.

17. Retrieved May 13, 2015, from http://obamacarefacts.com/vision-insurance/. Retrieved May 19, 2015, from http://www.aoa.org/newsroom/health-reform-offers-better-childrens-vision-care-in-the-us?sso=y.

18. Retrieved May 6, 2015, from http://ophthalmologytimes.modernmedicine.com/ophthalmologytimes/content/many-children-today-lack-good-vision-care?page=full.

19. Mozlin, Poverty, Neurodevelopment and Vision, 71–74.

20. Retrieved May 19, 2015, from http://www.visionandhealth.org/documents/child_vision_report.pdf.

21. Retrieved September 3, 2015, from https://visionhelp.files.wordpress.com/2013/06/vision-learning-obena-2013-wash-state-public-health.pdf.

22. Orfield, A. (2007). *Eyes for Learning: Preventing and Curing Vision-Related Learning Problems*. Lanham, Maryland: Rowman & Littlefield; p. 90.

23. Orfield, *Eyes for Learning*, 230.

REFERENCES

BOOKS

Appelbaum, Stanley A., and Ann M. Hoopes. *Eye Power*. Dr. Stanley A. Appelbaum and Ann M. Hoopes, 2009.

Barry, Susan R. *Fixing My Gaze*. New York: Basic Books, 2009.

Bennett, Sara, and Nancy Kalish. *The Case Against Homework*. New York: Crown Publishers, 2006.

Benoit, Robin, with Jillian Benoit. *Jillian's Story*. Berkeley, California: The Small Press, 2010.

———. *Dear Jillian*. Berkeley, California: The Small Press, 2013.

Crain, William. *Reclaiming Childhood*. New York: Henry Holt and Company, 2003.

Dennison, Paul E., and Gail E. Dennison. *Brain Gym: Simple Activities for Whole Brain Learning*. Ventura, California: Edu-Kinesthetics, 1992.

Gardner, Howard. *Multiple Intelligences: The Theory in Practice*. New York: Basic Books, 1993.

Hannaford, Carla. *Smart Moves: Why Learning Is Not All In Your Head*. Salt Lake City, Utah: Great River Books, 2005.

Hellerstein, Lynn. *See It. Say It. Do It!* Centennial, Colorado: HiClear Publishing, 2010.

Johnson, Katie. *Red Flags for Elementary Teachers*. Denver, Colorado: Tendril Press, 2015.

Kranowitz, Carol. *The Out-of-Sync Child*. New York: The Penguin Group, 2005.

Kranowitz, Carol, and Joye Newman. *Growing an In-Sync Child*. New York: Penguin Group, 2010.

Louv, Richard. *Last Child in the Woods*. Chapel Hill, North Carolina: Algonquin Books of Chapel Hill, 2008.

Orfield, Antonia. *Eyes for Learning: Preventing and Curing Vision-Related Learning Problems*. Lanham, Maryland: Rowman & Littlefield, 2007.

Pica, Rae. *What if Everybody Understood Child Development? Straight Talk About Bettering Education and Children's Lives*. Thousand Oaks, California: Corwin Press, 2015.

Seiderman, Arthur S., and Steven E. Marcus. *20/20 Is Not Enough: The New World of Vision*. New York: Alfred A. Knopf, 1989.

WEBSITES

http://www.visionandlearning.org
http://www.optometrists.org
http://www.visionhelp.org
http://www.pressvision.com
http://www.allaboutvision.com/parents/learning.htm
http://www.covd.org(find a practitioner here)
http://www.oepf.org
http://www.pavevision.org
http://www.concussionproject.com
http://www.nora.cc
http://www.devdelay.org
http://www.braingym.org
http://www.visionandhealth.org/documents/child_vision_report.pdf
https://visionhelp.files.wordpress.com/2013/06/vision-learning-obena-2013-wash-state-public-health.pdf

INTERVIEWS

Cotter, S. February 5, 2015. Interviewer: W. Rosen.
Crain, W. March 30, 2015. Interviewer: W. Rosen.
Guddemi, M. February 6, 2015. Interviewer: W. Rosen.
Haines, J. May, 2015. Interviewer: W. Rosen.
Harris, P. 2014. Interviewer: W. Rosen.
Hellerstein, L. January 22, 2015. Interviewer: W. Rosen.
Hillier, C. May 26, 2015. Interviewer: W. Rosen.
Johnson, K. April 29, 2015. Interviewer: W. Rosen.
Kranowitz, C. March 26, 2015. Interviewer: W. Rosen.
Lenart, T. May 20, 2015. Interviewer: W. Rosen.
Lyons, S. January 22, 2015. Interviewer: W. Rosen.
Montecalvo, B. February 4, 2015. Interviewer: W. Rosen.
Mozlin, R. May 22, 2015. Interviewer: W. Rosen.
Newman, J. April 13, 2015. Interviewer: W. Rosen.
Padula, W. V. March 3, 2015. Interviewer: W. Rosen.
Patel, K. January 12, 2015. Interviewer: W. Rosen.
Press, L., March 10, 2015. Interviewer: W. Rosen.
Scheiman, M. 2008. Interviewer: W. Rosen
Tamm, L. January 23, 2015. Interviewer: W. Rosen.
Torgerson, N. May 11, 2015. Interviewer: W. Rosen.
Valenti, C. May 12, 2015. Interviewer: W. Rosen.
Watt, J. February 4, 2015. Interviewer: W. Rosen.
Wesler, J. April 20, 2015. Interviewer: W. Rosen.

INDEX

Abeles, Vicki, 121
aberrant behavior, of children, 93
achievement, of children, 70
action system, 118
acuity. *See* visual acuity
AD/HD, 19, 21, 34, 67, 81, 135
Affordable Care Act, 103, 137
age group ranges, for sleep, 76–77
Alliance for Childhood, 36
Almon, Joan, 36
amblyopia, 105
American Academy of Optometry, 107
American Academy of Pediatrics, 37
American Educational Research
    Association, 73
American Optometric Association, 4, 29,
    58, 61, 103, 107
Ameri-Corps Child Vision Project, 138
Ames, Louise Bates, 129
Anderson, Daniel R., 37
Andrew, VT for, 160
anxiety, of children, 69, 76
Applebaum, Stan, 34
astigmatism, 5
auditory learning, 123
Australasian College of Behavioural
    Optometry, 60
automaticity, 10, 12
awareness, of vision-related learning
    problems, 19, 145

balance, with children, 80, 81, 88, 129
Barry, Susan, 104–105
Basch, Charles, 133–134
Becky, VT for, 156
behavior. *See* aberrant behavior, of
    children; criminal behavior, visual
    deficits and; neuromotor behavior
    patterns
behavioral optometrists, 53–54, 71, 83, 84,
    132, 142
behavioral optometry, 45–48, 50, 66, 104
behavior problems, with vision-related
    learning problems, 26–27, 92
Bennett, Sara, 73
Benoit, Jillian, 105
Benoit, Robin, 105
Better Vision Institute, 4
bilateral integration, 8
binocularity, 6, 24, 25–26, 143
blinking, 3, 74
blurry vision, of Jenny, 159
bodily/kinesthetic intelligence, 125–126
body: learning outcomes and, 85–87. *See
    also* mind-body connection
brain: concussions of, 38–42; information
    in, 119; nerve impulses and, 109;
    plasticity and malleability of, 37–38;
    vision skills and, 32–33, 88
brain, visual system and: imaging of, 13;
    mind's eye and, 12, 13; neurological
    pathways in, 12; visualization with, 10,

ABOUT THE AUTHOR

Over the course of her diverse career as an educator, **Wendy Beth Rosen** has taught preschool through high school students in public and private schools, as well as in informal educational frameworks. A proponent of innovation in the field of education, she has developed numerous curriculum resources on a variety of educational topics and has facilitated professional development workshops for teachers and administrators. Most recently, Wendy has designed a workshop and supplementary handbook about metacognition for high school and college students. She continues to apply her expertise about vision-related learning problems to the advancement of education and advocacy efforts.